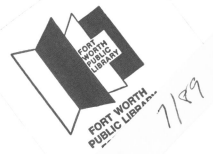

ALPHA

—&—

OMEGA

ALPHA
—&—
OMEGA

ETHICS AT THE
FRONTIERS OF
LIFE AND DEATH

A PORTABLE STANFORD BOOK

ERNLÉ W.D. YOUNG

ADDISON-WESLEY PUBLISHING COMPANY, INC.

Reading, Massachusetts   Menlo Park, California   New York
Don Mills, Ontario   Wokingham, England   Amsterdam   Bonn
Sydney   Singapore   Tokyo   Madrid   San Juan

This edition is published by arrangement with the Stanford Alumni Association.

Library of Congress Cataloging-in-Publication Data

Young, Ernlé W. D.
    Alpha and Omega: ethics at the frontiers of life and death / by Ernlé Young.
        p.   cm. — (A Portable Stanford book)
    Includes index.
    ISBN 0–201–18199–1
    1. Medical ethics. I. Title.
R724.Y68   1989
174′.2 — dc19   88-34909
                                                    CIP

Jacket design by Lynn Breslin
Set in 11-point Palatino by Terry Robinson & Co., Inc., San Francisco, CA

ABCDEFGHIJ–DO–89
First printing, January 1989

Contents

Preface

The writing of this book has been but part of an ongoing process of formulating, propounding, and revising my ideas on important issues. Typically, the process would begin as I prepared myself to hold forth in the classroom or the lecture hall; sometimes it would start as I thought about an article I had undertaken to produce. The process would continue as others responded critically to what I had said or written. Invariably, the criticisms offered were helpful, compelling me to refine or reformulate the positions I had outlined. You, the reader, are now invited to become involved in this process. It is to be hoped that you, in reading this book, and I, in receiving your response to it, will mutually benefit.

My acknowledgments, therefore, begin with my students and with those who have either listened to what I have said, or read what I have written, and reacted to it. You have been my teachers, and I am grateful. Miriam Miller, my editor, has been part of this process. Her critical comments have been astute and incisive. I have come to respect her judgment and competence. With affection, I express my thanks to her; she has made this a better book than it would have been without her wise suggestions. Gayle Hemenway, the talented production coordinator of Portable Stanford, and Jeffrey Whitten, the remarkably creative book designer, have brought this book to the form in which it appears before you; to both of them I am indebted. And I owe a debt of gratitude to you, the reader. In this age of electronic communication, readers of serious books are a vanishing breed. Thank you for taking the time to struggle with weighty matters and, in anticipation, for affording me your critical reflection on what I have written!

Linda Judd, word processor par excellence, our office manager, a devoted colleague, and my trusted friend, has been both indispensable and indefatigable in helping to produce the manuscript. For this, as for so many other things, I am deeply indebted to her. Thanks are due, also, to Joe Civetta, M.D., editor, and the J.B. Lippincott Company for permission to include in this volume elements of my chapter in the textbook, *Critical Care*; and to James Bopp, Jr., J.D., editor, and to the publishers of *Issues in Law and Medicine*, for their permission to reproduce in this book substantial parts of an article which first appeared in their journal.

Not least, I owe more than I could ever adequately express to Margaret, my wife; Heather, Andrew, Jenny, and Timothy, our children; and Peggy, my mother. Each in their own way has enabled me to become who I am and to do what I do. They have my enduring thanks and my unbounded love. This book is gladly dedicated to them.

Atherton, California
September, 1988

1

Grappling at the Frontiers Is Not "Playing God"

The phrase "playing God" is commonly bandied about with reference to many of the topics to be addressed in this book. To intervene in the evolutionary process through so-called genetic engineering techniques, or in the natural mode of reproduction by means of some of the technologies now in use to resolve problems of infertility, is defined as playing God. To make decisions about whether babies or adults live or die is also defined as playing God. To consider helping someone who is terminally ill and in unmitigable pain to commit suicide is sometimes labeled playing God. So, too, is making resource allocation decisions, the consequences of which are that some will live and others will die. And, of course, jokes abound about physicians playing God and about God playing Doctor. Occasionally, these are told even by reputable writers on ethics.[1]

Although the expression playing God is employed loosely, without precise definition, it seems to connote two complementary points of view. One is that decisions about matters of life and death are the prerogative of God, not of human beings. The other is that for human beings to assume the burden of making these decisions exhibits the hubris of overreaching, of transgressing certain divinely imposed limits. Briefly, I wish to challenge these suppositions.

It strikes me as odd that the allegation of playing God is one brought almost exclusively against members of the medical profession. Lawyers who make arguments that result in juries convicting people of first-degree murder and judges who sentence such people to die in electric chairs or by lethal injection are not commonly charged with playing God. The engineers who design bridges, the contractors who build them, and the inspectors who certify them as safe are not accused of playing God if such structures later collapse and the people traveling upon them at the time are swept away to a watery death. Nor do we reproach military commanders for playing God when in times of war they give orders that lead to the death of some of the men under their command or, worse, of innocent civilians. Why matters of life and death in the medical arena alone should invite such implied censure is puzzling.

Perhaps this simply indicates the extent to which the average American has been willing to place on a pedestal anyone practicing medicine. Even if this idolatrous attitude is inexorably giving way to more realistic expectations of those engaged in the healing arts, it is still prevalent. Consequently, when physicians do things the results of which are untoward, the ordinary person's sense of having been let down is disproportionately greater than when failures in the legal system, the construction industry, or the military come to light. Physicians' decisions are not seen as honest attempts to make the best possible choices in difficult circumstances. It is assumed that doctors manifest the desire, mostly hidden from view, to usurp divine prerogatives; that they, of all professionals, are uniquely guilty of arrogance and conceit. Such is the fate of the clay-footed whom we place on pedestals!

If intervening in the medical arena to change nature's course is considered playing God, where are we to stop—or start? Whenever we vaccinate a child, receive a booster tetanus injection, or donate blood for transfusion purposes, we are interfering in the way events would unfold if left to themselves. If such activities do not warrant accusations of playing God, why then should decisions about withdrawing or withholding ventilators and antibiotics, or intervening at the genetic level rather than surgically, chemically, or radiologically? It is not clear where the boundary lies between warranted and unwarranted intrusion into the natural order.

More particularly, objections must be raised to the assumptions that appear to underlie the notion of playing God. The first is that life and death decisions are the prerogative of God, not of human beings. Such phrases as "his time had come," "her number was up," or "it was meant to be" all express and reinforce the popular belief that it is God alone who ought to determine who is to live and who is to die, and when, where, and how. Yet this belief is contradicted by the fact that all of us are making life and death choices every day of our lives: decisions about what we eat; what kind of work we do and where we do it; how we get to and from work and at what speed; what habits we indulge (cigarette smoking rather than exercising, as an example); what recreational activities we pursue (hang gliding is surely riskier than stamp collecting!) and what life-style in general we will follow. Any and all of these factors have a demonstrable effect both on longevity and on morbidity. Whose prerogative is it, then, to make life and death determinations? We talk as though it were God's; we act as though it were our own!

A second assumption to be critically examined is that for human beings to assume the burden of making life and death decisions is to display hubris, to manifest sure signs of overreaching, of trespassing beyond divinely imposed limits. Unconsciously, all of us are continually making decisions that have a bearing on how long and how well we shall live.[2] We accept this as normal. But we become concerned when physicians consciously decide that certain medical interventions are inappropriate, take steps to withhold or withdraw them, and death ensues. Perhaps the problem resides in our unwillingness to recognize the full range of our unconscious or automatic choices, day by day, and our proclivity for regarding as decisions only those that are made consciously and which are, in the nature of things, often more onerous and far-reaching. Since the stakes are so high in medicine, the charge of hubris is readily invited, however unfair this may be.

The myth of the Garden of Eden provides a rationale for thinking that God once set absolute limits to human choice: "You may eat from every tree in the garden, but not from the tree of the knowledge of good and evil; for on the day that you eat from it, you shall certainly die."[3] Adam and Eve chose to trespass beyond this boundary. But the rest of the story makes it clear that this was not their cardinal offense. Their principal lapse was that of failing to take responsibility for the decision they had made. The man blames the woman for what he had done: "The woman you gave me for a companion, she gave me fruit from the tree and I ate it."[4] And the woman excuses herself by shifting culpability to the serpent: "The serpent tricked me, and I ate."[5] Then follows not death but, more mercifully, the expulsion from the garden. The consequences—alienation of human life from other forms of life, woman's travail in childbearing, and the need to work in order to live—are all depicted as divine punishments for human irresponsibility. But these are the very aspects of the human predicament for which the myth had been devised to provide an explanation!

Human beings are called upon to take responsibility for the choices they make, for the way they use their freedom. This is the conclusion to be reached from an unbiased reading of the Genesis story—not that there is some divinely imposed and quite arbitrary limit to human inquiry. As autonomous moral agents, we are free to intervene in natural processes. For the most part, we have tended to use this freedom for the benefit and betterment of the human condition, although environmentalists, for example, rightly draw attention to the disastrous results of some of our interventions. In inventing and employing various forms of transportation and constructing the highways, bridges, and airports they require; in developing and deploying various kinds of medications as remedies for our ailments; in purifying water and piping it into our homes and buildings; in discovering, generating, and harnessing electricity so that it serves us in thousands of ways in daily life, we have attempted to improve our standard of living over that of our forebears.

Concomitant with the choices we have made to enter into hitherto uncharted territory, there has been the dawning, if reluctant and sometimes belated, recognition that it is our duty to take responsibility for the forces we have unleashed, using them wisely and well, for the common good. Where we have failed to do this—and our human failures have been many, as the fate of the cities of Hiroshima and Nagasaki, of the ozone layer, and of certain now-extinct species of fauna and flora remind us—we have had, and still have, to discover a way back from destructive to more fruitful consequences. The way back may be long, arduous, and painful, as the history of actual and attempted strategic arms limitation agreements attests. The penalty for not finding it may, in fact, be the annihilation of life on this planet as we know it. Yet searching for solutions is in itself indicative of our resolve to take responsibility for our human choices. As such, it exemplifies human integrity rather than superhuman arrogance.

It is of the essence of the *humanum* to be endowed with freedom. Obviously, our freedom is limited by genetic as well as environmental factors. You and I are not free to be two rather than five or six feet tall, nor to be twenty years younger, nor to be Latinos or Filipinos rather than American Indians or Anglos, or vice versa. Similarly, those millions who are starving in Ethiopia or Madagascar are not free to belong to affluent Europe, rather than impoverished Africa. But it is also our unending task as humans to learn to exercise what real freedom we have, individually and collectively, responsibly and well, for creative and constructive purposes, rather than for malevolent and destructive ends. As we assume this duty and begin to succeed at it, so we become more fully and truly human. So we grow in stature in ways that would never have been possible had we not been willing to risk going beyond imagined and arbitrary limits on our capacity to choose or decide.

As the following case makes clear, the patient and her social worker together made a decision which resulted in the patient's death, as she wished her death to occur. In doing this, neither of them was playing God; both were being responsibly human.

Mr. and Mrs. Bengt Bjorgsen were 86 and 84 years of age, respectively. Mrs. Bjorgsen had chronic obstructive pulmonary disease (COPD). They were immigrants who had realized the American dream. They had themselves built the house they lived in and had seen their children, grandchildren, and great grandchildren play and grow to maturity within the warm environment they had been able to provide. They had vowed to each other that they would stay in this home until they were parted by death. In recent years, the upkeep and maintenance of the house had become more difficult and burdensome. Not only was their property falling into disrepair, they themselves were beginning to look increasingly unkempt. From time to time their neighbors would call Adult Protective Services to "intervene," since the Bjorgsen children had by now moved away from the immediate area.

Mrs. Bjorgsen developed rectal cancer and came into the hospital for surgery; a colostomy was performed on her. While his wife was in the hospital, Mr. Bjorgsen had a myocardial infarction and died unexpectedly. In the meantime, Mrs. Bjorgsen was to have been discharged from the hospital— somewhat prematurely, since the amount allocated for her care by Medicare had been used up. She could afford to stay for only three or four days in the skilled nursing facility to which her caregivers wanted to refer her because they believed she needed care 24 hours a day. Since Medicare would not pay for convalescent care, she was adamant in wanting to return to her own home instead, thus conserving what savings she had and honoring her promise to her deceased husband. Her doctors and nurses were equally insistent in proclaiming that she could not manage to live by herself and needed skilled nursing care.

At this point, Mrs. Bjorgsen's social worker chose to become her advocate. Insisting that her client's values—her promise to her late husband, her fierce independence, her unwillingness to become a financial burden to her children—had to be honored, the social worker took the necessary steps to enable Mrs. Bjorgsen to return to her abode. She arranged for nurses to call on her three times a week and provided oxygen for Mrs. Bjorgsen in her own home. Mrs. Bjorgsen went home content and was adequately cared for at minimal expense. Two weeks after returning home, she died peacefully.

To address seriously the ethical issues on the frontiers of life and death presented in this book does not, in my view, fall into the category of playing God. To go even further, I am unconvinced that such a category exists at all. The crucial question is not about limits to human inquiry and action, but rather about how responsibly to use what freedom we have. We shall attempt to address this question in relation to medicine and the life sciences in general, with a particular focus on issues arising at the beginnings and endings of life. It is to be hoped that the answers proposed will be regarded not as further examples of hubris, but rather as a modest contribution to facilitating our becoming whom we were created to be.

2

Medico-Moral Quandaries

Donald was born with cystic fibrosis, an ultimately fatal lung disease. Most cystic fibrosis patients succumb to this genetic malady in their late teens or early twenties. Donald lived until he was thirty-nine. For most of his life, he had been treated at Children's Hospital at Stanford. Now his lungs were so inelastic, so hard and rigid, that if he were to survive, even in the short term, he would have to be placed on a breathing machine for the first time in the course of his long struggle against debilitating disease. This was the background to his being brought into the intensive care unit at Stanford Hospital.

Shortly after his admission, Sibyl, who had nursed him during his many admissions to Children's Hospital, fallen in love with him, and become engaged to marry him, came to my office. She wanted me to visit Donald for two reasons: one had to do with an ethical issue; the other reflected a pastoral concern. The ethical issue was that Donald did not want to be kept alive on a breathing machine. He had been fiercely independent all his life and had lived as fully and normally as his disease would allow. He was unwilling to become dependent on a machine for his very survival at this late stage in the game. Yet his doctor, a pediatrician who had been treating him since he was a teenager and who still thought of him as a youngster rather than as a mature man, was having difficulty in letting go of his patient and acceding to Donald's wishes to be allowed to die naturally and peacefully. He wanted to make one last-ditch attempt to rescue him. Hence there was a conflict between Donald's autonomous choice and his primary physician's beneficent impulse. This was the dilemma Sibyl wanted me to help resolve.

Her concern was that Donald should then be enabled to have a good death.

The time had arrived when Donald's cystic fibrosis could no longer be kept in check. Sibyl wanted me to support him emotionally and counsel him spiritually throughout the dying process so that death, when it came, would be dignified and serene.

I readily responded to Sibyl's requests and at once began to establish relationships with both Donald and his physicians. What she was asking of me, after all, is precisely what I, as chaplain to the medical center and as the hospital's ethics consultant, am there to provide.

Stories like Donald's make it possible, and necessary, for me to write this book. It is written for the general reader, with or without a medical background. In recent years, several scholarly texts on biomedical ethics have appeared. For the most part, these are designed to benefit specialists in the field rather than a lay audience. Other than newspaper and magazine articles and special television programs, little on the subject of biomedical ethics is directly accessible to the public. There is an unmet need awaiting attention. The present work represents an attempt to meet this need in a way that will be both informed and intelligible.

My concern for these issues is augmented by my experience. For the last fourteen years, I have taught medical ethics to medical students, undergraduates, and graduate students from disciplines other than medicine at Stanford University. My own academic expertise enables me to understand and speak the various languages of theology, philosophy, and medicine—the three branches of knowledge which together have contributed to the evolution of bioethics as a field of research and reflection.

Additionally, as chaplain to the Stanford University Medical Center, one of my primary responsibilities is to provide emotional support and spiritual counsel to those who are confronted by life-threatening illnesses, sudden accidents, or imminent death. This is a service performed by all who work in the chaplaincy department, irrespective of the religious or denominational affiliation, or lack thereof, of those who call upon us. In large measure, spiritual needs transcend religious preferences. They have to do with the existential concerns of faith—that life is ultimately meaningful; of hope—that beyond death there is new life; and of love—that, in the end, loving oneself, loving others, and being loved by them matter more than anything else.

Another crucial aspect of my work is that of consulting on the bioethical issues which emerge constantly in the clinical setting. Clinical concerns may be raised either by caregivers—physicians, house officers, registered nurses, or third- and fourth-year medical students; or by those on the receiving end of medical care—patients and family members. As chair of the Hospital Ethics Committee, recently instituted by the chief of staff, one of my tasks is to implement its mandate. The topics about which I write are not merely of academic interest. They are matters which confront me day by day.

What are these ethical problems?

A biochemist friend is on the verge of identifying genetic markers for a whole series of devastating diseases: cystic fibrosis, certain types of breast cancer, schizophrenia, and possibly Alzheimer's, among others. He anticipates that within the next decade genetic fingerprints for most major diseases will have been found on the DNA chain, making possible the diagnosis *in utero* of illnesses that normally manifest themselves only in later life. He worries about who should have access to this information once it becomes available: the pregnant women carrying fetuses identified as having a potential disease? the affected children, as soon as it is possible for the import of a diagnosis to be understood? And, he asks, should these findings be included in the medical record, thus providing future health insurers or employers access to them?

A postdoctoral fellow in maternal-fetal health, with a slightly different perspective, is exercised by the same issue. Although she performs abortions, regarding abortion as an often tragic necessity, she does so with reluctance. She is raising children of her own and feels her child-rearing role to be in conflict with that of abortionist. She wonders what effect the new DNA assays will have on the practice of abortion. It is one thing to abort seriously defective fetuses. It is another to abort because of diseases that are not incompatible with a good quality of life for twenty, thirty, forty, fifty, or more years. If even treatable genetic abnormalities constitute grounds for terminating a pregnancy, it is unlikely that any of us would have survived, for in one respect or another, each of us deviates slightly from the genetic "norm," whatever that may be thought to be.

A colleague, a faculty member in the Department of Obstetrics/Gynecology, has recently instituted a program of *in vitro* fertilization designed to alleviate some of the problems of infertility. He has been approached by the director of a nationwide surrogacy agency, who wishes to enlist him and his fertility program in the commercial surrogate motherhood business. My colleague wrestles with this issue because of a perceived conflict between medicine as a service and medicine for profit and then consults with me. What should he do?

Another faculty member, a prominent neonatologist, continually struggles with the morally problematic endeavor of aggressively treating extremely low-birthweight premature infants, in the 500–750-gram range—little more than a pound to a pound and a half—at enormous cost (on average, scores of thousands of dollars) and with uncertain benefits for the infants themselves. Only 25 percent survive newborn intensive care, and of these, only 70 percent turn out to be normal. He wonders whether the funds expended in his unit would do more long-term good if invested in providing preventive medical care to pregnant women.

A registered nurse in the medical/surgical intensive care unit invites an ethical consultation about an 84-year-old patient who is on a ventilator because of chronic emphysema and is only marginally competent. The patient's daughter claims that her father once signed a "living will," stating that if ever he found himself in the kind of situation he is now in he would want all aggressive therapy to be withdrawn. The daughter communicates this to the attending physician. The physician, believing that his patient's problems are not yet irreversible, is unwilling to go along with the daughter's request to withdraw ventilatory support so that her father may have "a natural and peaceful death." The nurse finds herself torn between two opposing points of view. How can this dilemma be resolved?

A husband whose wife is terminally ill with advanced cancer approaches the physician taking care of her with a request that her dying be hastened with a lethal injection. The wife is in unmitigable pain. The cancer has now spread to her bones, and every time she is moved another bone breaks. She herself had asked previously to be helped to die when the disease made life intolerable. Yet for the physician to comply with the husband's request would be a criminal act. In the state of California, the penalty for assisting someone to commit suicide is up to five years' imprisonment. The physician weighs his moral convictions against the legal constraints to which he is subject. He invites an ethical consultation in order to clarify and rank his obligations to his patient, his profession, and himself.

As a final example, an internist seeks an ethical consultation about a 29-year-old woman, a diabetic and an intravenous drug abuser who has access to a plentiful supply of needles because of the insulin injections she has to give herself daily. For the second time she has tested positive for the human immunodeficiency virus (HIV). She had also been found to be HIV positive six months earlier, but this piece of information is by law disallowed in the medical record. Although she has had a boyfriend for the past two or three months, she is and has been sexually active with others as well as with him. According to her own testimony, she never uses any kind of protection. What can the internist do to safeguard her sexual and needle contacts from possibly being infected with the AIDS virus? Although AIDS is a reportable disease, as are syphilis and gonorrhea, exposure to the human immunodeficiency virus (HIV), which is typically but not invariably a precursor to AIDS, is not. Yet the woman's behavior is potentially lethal. The confidentiality and privacy to which this patient has a right are obviously in conflict with the common good.

These are the sorts of medico-moral quandaries that I address in the course of my work, both in the hospital setting and in teaching biomedical ethics. Each of the examples provided corresponds with a chapter on the same topic in Parts Two and Three of this book.

At the outset, the reader is entitled to an indication of how I approach such problems. In the next chapter, the question of methodology will be discussed in more depth and detail. At this juncture, however, there may already be some nagging suspicions in the reader's mind: are not chaplains prone to attack moral issues dogmatically, moralistically, even judgmentally? After all, religious leaders are often at the forefront of the anti-abortion movement, of the crusade against homosexuality, or of the opposition to the various right-to-die initiatives. Why should *this* chaplain be trusted to deal reasonably and objectively with ethical conundrums? Should there be such concerns, they warrant a response.

I do, indeed, have my own religious convictions, which shape the values by which I try to live. I also find certain important moral principles embedded in the Christian tradition: principles like respect for persons, the foundation of our modern concern for *autonomy*; a commitment to *justice* which, in its distributive aspect, requires that we attempt to be evenhanded in allocating scarce resources; the call to act *beneficently*, as exemplified in the story of the man who went down from Jerusalem to Jericho and fell among robbers who beat him, stripped him, and left him half dead, being helped by a "good" Samaritan (Luke 10:25-37); and *nonmaleficence*, the duty not to harm even the enemy. Although it may not be generally known, these principles are also central to the Western medical tradition. At least two of them, *beneficence* and *nonmaleficence*, go back to about the fourth century B.C.

But there are two additional fundamental precepts which guide both my professional and my personal conduct. These inform what I do as a chaplain, as a consultant, and as a teacher. One is never to attempt to impose my own values on others. To do this would betray a lack of respect for the convictions and commitments by which others live. The other is to appeal to reason, not to any special revelation, in any ethical argument I might want to make on the basis of broad moral principles and cherished values. Because I consider these scruples so indispensable for both academic and religious freedom, I frequently discover myself to be at odds with other religious leaders, whether they be Protestant literalists, Roman Catholics seeking refuge in supposedly infallible hierarchical pronouncements, Jewish ultra-conservatives, or Muslim fundamentalists.

The reader need not be concerned that this book is a pretext for some thinly veiled evangelical enterprise or that it will claim to settle complex moral questions, once and for all, by appeal to revelation from some supernatural authority. Where necessary, I will state my own values as well as the principles I consider pertinent to the discussion; always, the implicit invitation to the reader will be to do the same. The arguments made will have to bear scrutiny and be defensible in a public forum, where others are at liberty to contend or concur with them. Any solution one proposes to a vexing moral quandary represents nothing more than the best one can come up with at the time after struggling with it honestly. That is not to say that with fresh light on the subject, newer information, or more accurate data, one might not decide differently. If this book stimulates thought and debate about even a few of the issues it addresses, then its writing will have been worth the effort. It is the ongoing consideration of important topics that matters, not necessarily one's own position on any one of them at a given time.

It took about a week to overcome the ethical impasse between Donald and his pediatrician. What the pediatrician wanted was to offer Donald a bronchopulmonary lavage: under general anesthesia, first one lung and then, a week later, the other would be washed out with a saline solution. Although this procedure was popular ten years ago, when it was thought to offer promise of treating cystic fibrosis, most modern medical centers have by now abandoned it. It held only the slimmest prospect of prolonging the patient's

01370 5741

life without need for a breathing machine. Donald eventually decided to take this chance with the understanding that if the attempt was unsuccessful, he would be granted his wish to be allowed to die naturally. The first broncho-pulmonary lavage was done. Unfortunately, the net effect was to make Donald worse rather than better. Somehow, as a result of it, he became infected with a virulent pneumonia. There was by this time no thought of even attempting to wash out his second lung.

Donald died about two weeks after Sibyl had first come into my office. His dying represented a triumph of the human spirit. Marked by courage, joy, and peace, it was remarkable for the loving, open communication between him, on the one hand, and, on the other, Sibyl, his parents, his doctors and nurses, and his chaplain. His memorial service was an unforgettable celebration of the way in which Donald had lived and died. Moving final tributes were offered to his indomitable will to survive, to his unquenchable zest for life, and to his steadfast refusal to enter into the expected role of a sick person. With felt-tipped pens we wrote on helium balloons our prayers and wishes for Donald, now liberated for new life beyond death. On a breathtakingly beautiful spring day we released the balloons and watched them soar upward. As they floated upward, they lifted our spirits with them.

3

Ethical Issues
in Medicine

J ohn James is a third-year surgical resident at a major medical center.
His principal interest is in cardiac surgery, a field which includes,
among other things, heart-valve replacements, coronary artery bypass
grafts, the repair of such things as aneurysms and "holes in the heart," heart
and heart-lung transplantations, and temporary artificial heart
implantations.

A patient, Arthur G., is referred to him from a nearby state institution
for the profoundly mentally disabled. Arthur, 35 years old, was born with
Down's syndrome, with complications that included a congenital heart malformation. His parents did not wish to be "burdened" with a less-than-
normal child; hence his lifelong institutionalization. As the years unfolded,
Arthur's IQ, which for people with Down's syndrome could be anything
between 40 and 70 on the Stanford-Binet scale, turned out to be at the lowest
possible end of the spectrum. Incapable of any kind of relationship with other
human beings, Arthur's capacity for autonomous self-determination was
zero. His congenital heart defect had become incompatible with continued
survival and required immediate surgical intervention.

For cardiac surgeons, Arthur's medical problems were simply correctable.
Unfortunately, however, no one could hope to remedy his neurological deficits. Despite the fact that for someone like Arthur death might be a release
from a life of questionable quality, state law requires that everything possible,
medically or surgically, be done for institutionalized mental patients. Ought
John James to set in motion a process that will lead to the surgery being
performed and Arthur's life being saved? Or ought he, on humanitarian and
compassionate grounds, decide that the surgery, however technically feasible,

is contraindicated and thus allow Arthur a gentle exit from a life most of us would deem to be not worth living? The first option is legally safe. The second might be morally preferable, yet be legally hazardous. What ought John James to do? And why?

———

Sheila W., 32 years of age, has had a double mastectomy. Physically, she is doing well after this disfiguring surgery. Mentally and emotionally, she is in turmoil. Her anger and bitterness are manifest. Five years ago, her husband, from whom she is now divorced, prompted her to do something she now regrets profoundly. A man obviously nurtured on Playboy and Penthouse magazines, by both verbal and nonverbal communications he constantly made her feel that her breasts were too small. Sheila went to a state where silicone breast implantations are legal to have her breasts enlarged by a plastic surgeon. Unfortunately, as is frequently the case, the silicone used for breast implantations subsequently turned bad. Deep infection set in. Five years later, Sheila had no recourse but to have a double, total mastectomy.

Now, after the fact, she was wise—as she had not been five years earlier. Too late she was asking, "How ought that plastic surgeon to have handled my case, when first I went to him? Ought he to have done what for him was financially remunerative and for me was emotionally promising, to implant liquid silicone into both my breasts, the medical risks of this procedure notwithstanding? Or ought he to have urged me to find a therapist who could help me cope with my problem of self-esteem, or advised both me and my husband to seek counseling—at some financial loss to himself?" These tormenting questions raise the issue of the ethical obligation of the responsible physician.

These questions from real life, posed in the first instance by John James, a physician, and in the second by Sheila W., a patient, bring to our attention more theoretical but related issues: How might one go about the process of making up one's mind in an ethically responsible way? How might one go about analyzing the arguments on either side of a controversial moral dilemma so as to identify inconsistencies, incongruities, or faulty logic? How might one go about formulating normative proposals of one's own? What part does reason play in a moral decision? And feelings? These questions invite reflection on the process of making an ethical decision and take us to the heart of the subject to which this chapter is devoted. There are five steps constituent to the process of making moral decisions.

Identifying the Central Problem or Problems

Frequently what is presented as an ethical problem turns out, on closer examination, to be a difficulty stemming from a breakdown in communication: physicians not communicating with nurses or with families, or one team of physicians not communicating with another. Sometimes what appears to be a dilemma in medical ethics may actually be a Gordian knot in the social or political arena. As examples, consider the predicament of a resident physician presented with an indigent person in need of medical attention in a hospital no longer providing care to those unable to pay for it. Or the quandary of a psychiatrist in charge of the one small (25-bed) locked facility in a county, with inadequate nursing staff, when presented with a psychopathic, disruptive, and dangerous patient.

Clearly, the central problem or problems must be identified: What are the cardinal issues in the case? Do they legitimately fall within the purview of medical ethics? Or do they have to do with matters of etiquette, poor communication, a breakdown in interpersonal relationships, or larger social ills? If there are a number of problems, how might they be ranked in order of importance?

Gathering Information from As Many Sources As Possible

To make decisions about moral dilemmas in medicine, we need to begin with accurate medical information. The importance of a right diagnosis and of the many technological diagnostic tools now available to physicians cannot be overemphasized in this regard. But we may not stop there. It is also necessary to acquire relevant data about the personal, social, economic, religious, and cultural context of the problem.

The values of the observer inevitably determine which facts are selected for scrutiny, as well as how they are interpreted and understood. But the gathering of facts from as wide a range of perspectives as possible provides a check and balance against an overly subjective selection and examination of the available evidence.

In order to arrive at a right diagnosis and to recommend appropriate treatment, the physician requires access to extensive privileged patient information. For the patient to provide personal data of the most intimate sort, he or she must trust the physician sufficiently to be assured that what is said within the confines of the consulting room will go no further.

Certain standards have evolved over the course of time that affect the kind of behavior patients look for in their physicians. It is expected that physicians will be truthful in communicating with those whom they treat and that they will respect the privacy and honor the confidentiality of patients in their care. Only for the most serious reasons, usually having to do with the well-being of others, may the standards of privacy and confidentiality be breached.[1] Only when they paternalistically decide that telling patients the truth will do more harm than good will physicians deviate from truthfulness as a norm. Such paternalism, however, is increasingly abhorrent to consumers of medical services in the United States, and beneficently motivated lying is steadily giving way to a more complete openness in the physician-patient relationship.

The significant place even nonmedical facts may have in the decision-making process is illustrated by the following story:

In the days before the human immunodeficiency virus (HIV) had been isolated and a test for HIV developed, one of the patients in the intensive care unit was a 25-year-old man who was running a high fever. His doctors were unable to identify either the source of an infection or any other reason for his feverishness. In the course of a pastoral conversation with him, this young man confided to me that he was both homosexual and highly promiscuous. He was concerned that God would reject and damn him because of his life-style. After offering him what reassurance I could on this score, I asked him whether he had told the physicians caring for him what he had divulged to me. He had not. Suspecting that his fever might indicate that he had AIDS (acquired immunodeficiency syndrome), I urged him to tell his doctors the facts that, until then, he had kept from everyone except his chaplain. With some diffidence, he agreed to do this. The information he went on to provide to his physicians led to a diagnosis of AIDS. Once this diagnosis had been made, the ethical question of the appropriateness of intensive care in the hospital rather than palliative care at home could be addressed. The upshot was that he eventually left the hospital and went home to die—surrounded by people who loved him.

The difficulty of acquiring accurate information is illustrated by the number of important issues on which the medical community itself has not yet reached agreement. A study published in the *New England Journal of Medicine* suggests that aspirin can effectively lower the risk of myocardial infarction; almost simultaneously, another study is published in *Lancet* in which contradictory conclusions are drawn. The

First Lady undergoes a mastectomy for breast cancer; at once, medical experts are divided over the appropriateness of this particular treatment *vis-à-vis* other less disfiguring and arguably equally efficacious alternatives.

A published study documents the correlation between high cholesterol levels and cardiovascular disease; a prominent cardiovascular surgeon disagrees with these findings in the light of his experience in having performed more than 15,000 open-heart surgeries; and pediatricians disagree about the implications of this study for modifications to the dietary recommendations for growing children. Even a practice as common as circumcision is contentious, with pros and cons vigorously propounded; the only agreement is that circumcision is painful to the infant, though probably far less painful for infants than it is for adults. The point is that acquiring factual information can be a long and laborious process, requiring constant reconsideration and revision of earlier hypotheses and opinions.

Identifying the Values Involved

Values enter into every decision we make, personally as well as collectively. These may be either unconsciously or consciousiy held. Ultimately, agreement about values may be impossible. Identifying those values that are in conflict in a given situation, however, may at least allow for agreement about where to disagree, and why.

Because, in the final analysis, values derive from metaphysical assumptions or beliefs about the essential nature of reality, they are typically espoused with emotion, even passion. Believing that the use of blood products is proscribed in the Scriptures, Jehovah's Witnesses typically are implacably opposed to blood transfusions, either for themselves or for their children. As those will know who have attempted to deal rationally with people committed to dogmatic religious tenets, intense feelings are evoked when these are at stake. Such emotions are quite foreign to the dispassionate approach that relies on reason alone. Yet they are equally part of the human constitution and, up to a point, ought to be accorded a legitimate place in the decision-making process.

It is one thing for adult Jehovah's Witnesses to refuse blood transfusions for themselves. It is a quite different matter when the refusal will affect the well-being of a child—either indirectly, since the child's primary caregiver may die as a result of her unwillingness to accept treatments involving blood products, or directly, when the parents act as proxy for the child requiring blood products and decline potentially life-giving interventions.

That the various participants in a discussion about a moral dilemma in medicine not only be both clear and honest about their own values, but also recognize and respect one another's, is essential. This will encourage the patient to begin to define for himself what is an acceptable quality of life. It will also permit the medical caregiver to determine what procedures are unacceptable in light of her values, such as prescribing enough medication to allow a terminally ill patient to commit suicide. Further, it will compel the decision maker to recognize the ways in which a society's values enter into choices made in the medical arena. That our own society allocates millions upon millions of dollars to the strategic defense initiative but not commensurate amounts to alleviating the plight of the homeless is indicative of our underlying values.

Determining the Rational Component in a Moral Decision

In the history of ethical theory, rational reflection has tended to focus on the principal elements in any action: the *motive* of the agent, the agent's *intention,* the *means* used by the agent to accomplish the act, and the *consequences* of the action.

- *Ethical theories of virtue*, which flourished until the Renaissance, when they went into eclipse, but are once again attracting increasing interest, concentrate on the agent's motives and intentions.

- *Teleological* or *consequentialist ethical systems*—from the Greek word TELOS, "end,"—of which utilitarianism is a prime example, shift the locus of concern to the consequences of an action.

- *Deontological theories of ethics*—from the Greek word DEON, "it is required" or "it is necessary,"—refer to the means used to accomplish an action, holding that means are intrinsically either right or wrong.

These terms require some explanation.

Ethics of Virtue

An ethical theory of virtue concentrates on the question, "How does one become a virtuous human being?" Implicit is the belief that right conduct will flow naturally from intrinsic goodness. Proponents of this approach to ethics thus advocate the inward look: a rigorous examination of motives, intentions, and aspirations, and an evaluation of these in the light of the highest personal and professional standards of the traditions in which one stands. It is a fact of life in our complex times that many of the problems we confront at the national and international levels are impervious to sheerly rational resolution. Our best hope may be to have leaders of genuine integrity, of authentic virtue, whose judgment about what is the right thing to do in any given situation may be trusted. Recent revelations about insider trading on Wall Street, sleazy behavior on the part of television evangelists, and plagiarism and philandering by prominent politicians point to a regrettable lack of virtue in many of those in positions of leadership. An ethics of virtue takes us back to the source of morality: purity of heart, clarity of spirit, and nobleness of mind.

Teleological or Consequentialist Ethics

A consequentialist approach to resolving moral dilemmas is (a) to imagine both the immediate and the long-term consequences of various alternative courses of action, (b) to weigh the immediate and long-range benefits and harms of each, and then choosing either (c) to act according to your findings or (d) to apply the appropriate rule so as to either maximize the benefits or minimize the harms for the greatest possible number.

Consequentialism is not without its difficulties. How are "harms" and "benefits" to be defined? Who is to do the defining? Once defined, how are immediate benefits to be weighed against long-term harms? On what basis? And what about the minority, those who do not fall into the category of "the greatest possible number"? A further concern is that consequentialism readily lends itself in our time to calculations of cost-effectiveness, whereby the results of actions are reduced almost entirely to financial profits or losses, causing the dollar sign to loom increasingly large in the decision-making process.

Despite these caveats, a consequentialist approach is a helpful way of attempting to resolve moral difficulties. It makes the moral agent responsible for thinking about and attempting to weigh the results of all the various possible courses of action. It also allows the moral agent freedom to choose among the alternatives. Freedom and responsibility are essential constituents of human behavior, and both are recognized and upheld in a consequentialist approach.

Deontological Ethics

A deontological ethics insists that certain things are inherently right or wrong. For instance, killing, deceiving, and stealing are wrong in and of themselves, and are therefore, *prima facie*, presumed to be impermissible. Being evenhanded or just in dealing with others, compassionate and respectful of their personhood and human dignity, are right and are typically required of us. Usually, the deontological approach determines the intrinsic rightness or wrongness of acts by appeal to revelation—for example, the Ten Commandments, the teachings of Jesus, or the Koran. Theological ethical systems have therefore been uniformly deontological rather than consequentialist. This means that, in a given situation, someone in the deontological tradition will hold, *a priori*, that certain actions are right or wrong and are thus required or prohibited regardless of the consequences. Withholding the truth of a diagnosis from a patient, for example, is wrong; full disclosure is required, even if the consequences are potentially devastating to the recipient.

Traditionally, medicine has been deontological in its approach to moral problems, and it has been guided by a few broad principles, rather than by multiple and rigid rules. It has upheld as principles such duties as *beneficence*, benefiting the patient—often associated with preserving life; *nonmaleficence*, doing no harm or alleviating suffering; and *justice*, treating people equitably.[2] Again, let us take these and an additional, more modern, principle, *autonomy*, one at a time.

> • *Beneficence* suggests that it is the primary duty of the physician to benefit the patient. Usually, this means attempting to preserve the patient's life. Preserving life has its roots in the Judaic element in our Judeo-Christian heritage. So fundamental is this principle that things otherwise prohibited by Jewish law must be set aside to preserve life. "Thus even though it is forbidden to mutilate a corpse, heart and kidney transplants as well as corneal grafting are permitted, provided of course that the utmost care is taken to be sure that the person whose body is being used for the purpose is really dead."[3]

• *Nonmaleficence*, the duty not to harm, is recognized in most deontological theories. It is an inescapable imperative in the Christian scriptures[4] honored, let it be said with some shame, more in the breach than in the observance! It is also associated with the medico-moral maxim, of uncertain origin, *primum non nocere*—above all, or first, do no harm. Of course, harm can be variously defined: for instance, in terms of death, disability, distress, or the deprivation of freedom and pleasure. However defined, harm has always to be weighed against hoped-for compensatory benefits. All medical interventions inflict some harm; one has only to observe a one-year-old being vaccinated to be aware of this! But usually, the inevitable harm is minimal and the ensuing benefits are many, although in certain settings, the intensive care unit, for example, the opposite may sometimes be true.

• *Justice*, as a guiding principle, is also fundamental to the Judeo-Christian tradition. One has only to remember the timeless words of Amos to be reminded of this: "Let justice roll on like a river and righteousness like an ever-flowing stream" (5:24). In its most basic terms, justice may be characterized as fairness. Fairness requires that we not do for some what we are unwilling or unable to do for all. To expend three-quarters of a million dollars on a single patient is one thing; to expend such colossal sums of money on all potential patients is manifestly impossible. We simply do not have the resources to do this. The principle of justice, then, presses upon us the questions: How can we fairly allocate what resources we have? How can we equitably distribute among the many claimants for services those relatively limited benefits that are available? Complicating the issue yet further is the fact that we do not yet have any consensus about what we mean by the term "justice."[5]

• *Autonomy*, which has only recently become central to the practice of medicine, is a principle whose origins can be traced back to the emphasis in the Judeo-Christian tradition on respect for persons.[6] Respecting the personhood of others requires that, as far as possible, we allow and enable them to be self-determining agents. Patients ought to be treated not as children by their physician-parents but as adults in adult-adult transactions. It requires that, as far as possible, patients be respected as equal partners in arriving at decisions affecting their own lives, and be encouraged to assume the concomitant responsibilities.

One of the weaknesses of a deontological approach to rational decision making is that it offers no guidance about what to do when principles come into conflict. Since no one principle is an absolute, how is the relative weight of principles opposed to one another to be assessed? When, for example, it is no longer possible both to attempt to preserve the life and to alleviate the suffering of a terminally ill patient, which maxim should take precedence, at what point, and why? At such junctures, I tend to adopt a consequentialist approach, for these are not mutually exclusive; neither do they require that insights derived from ethics of virtue be set aside. Each rational approach has its strengths and weaknesses. Each can usefully complement the others.

The Balancing of Personal and Professional Obligations

As a human being, the physician has constantly to weigh personal convictions against professional duties, deciding where the lines of compromise are to be drawn. As a citizen, the physician is obligated to obey the law and to work for change in society through the democratic process. As a professional, the physician has certain obligations: to the patient; to the parents or guardians of a patient who is a minor; to colleagues; to the hospital in which he has privileges; to third-party reimbursers, whether private, state, or federal; and to society at large, in reporting child abuse or infectious disease to the appropriate authorities, for example. The physician engaged in medical research may also feel a professional obligation both to a review board and to a large group of potential patients who are afflicted or likely to be afflicted with a particular disease.

At times, these various obligations may come into conflict. Withdrawing artificial life-support systems from an extensively and permanently brain-damaged patient who cannot be adjudged dead by the brain-death criterion may seem to a physician to be the right thing to do; nevertheless, it is illegal. If the physician follows her conscience, her obligation to be a law-abiding citizen will conflict with her duty to uphold the medico-moral principle of nonmaleficence. Enabling a pregnant teenager to have an abortion may meet the physician's obligation to benefit his patient; but when the teenager asks that information about this procedure be withheld from her parents, who may be paying the bill for the medical expenses, how does he simultaneously meet his obligation to the patient and to those legally and financially responsible for her?

The facts pertinent to the situation, the relevant values—the physician's, the patient's, the institution's, and society's—and serious rational reflection will all lead the physician to decide that her first duty lies in one direction rather than in others. This is the point of final commitment; hereafter, the chips must fall where they may.

In summary, the essential stages in arriving at a responsible moral decision in the area of biomedical ethics are: (1) isolating the central problem or problems; (2) accumulating a wide variety of pertinent facts; (3) identifying the values of the various parties involved in the decision-making process; (4) determining whether the reasoning is proceeding consequentially or deontologically; and (5) establishing the primary obligation of the medical caregiver in a given situation.

Seldom in the contemporary practice of medicine is the decision-making process confined to the individual physician and her patient. Inevitably, other actors become involved in playing out this drama. These may include family members, hospital administrators, registered nurses, consultant physicians in various specialties, house officers, social workers, chaplains, ethics consultants, and even legal counsel. This is why frequent disagreements are inevitable about the issue or issues being debated; about the relevant facts; about the values which are operative; about the proper way to proceed rationally; and about the overriding obligation or obligations of the caregiver.

John James must decide whether or not to initiate life-sustaining cardiac surgery for Arthur G., whose Down's syndrome is of such severity as to be incompatible with any appreciable quality of life. The problem could be identified as both medical and social. Arthur G. has obvious medical needs. Quite apart from his critical medical problems, it is questionable whether or not his life is worth living; yet he is being cared for in a societal institution which operates within well-defined legal constraints, including the requirement that everything possible be done medically for those in its charge. It is a fact that without the requisite surgery he will die. However, it is not possible to determine empirically what his experience of life is, and what it is worth to him; this can only be surmised.

In terms of values, the problem is simply stated: is death, which will follow if the surgery is not performed, preferable to the kind of life Arthur G. now experiences? Quality-of-life factors are easiest to include in the decision-making process and unequivocally acceptable when the patient is able to define these for himself; these considerations are most difficult and unsatisfactory when the patient is either incompetent or unconscious. Rationally, the deontological principles of preserving life and alleviating suffering appear to be in conflict, as Arthur G. may be suffering by being profoundly mentally incapacitated. The consequentialist weighing of alternatives is equally problematic: is his present life in the institution to be reckoned good or painful? If it is thought to be good, performing the surgery will assure its continuance; if it is deemed painful, performing the surgery would be contraindicated. What, then, is John James's obligation? To initiate or to withhold the cardiac surgery which alone can maintain Arthur G.'s continued physical existence?

This brings us to the point of decision. In my view, John James's obligation is to proceed to perform the cardiac surgery required to save the life of Arthur G. Although from the perspective of a normal observer Arthur G.'s quality of life seems abysmally poor, we have no factual evidence that this is how Arthur G. himself experiences it. Nor have we any indication that he is in pain—psychologically or emotionally. If it is difficult for the observer to value his life positively, it is even more difficult to demonstrate that Arthur G. would value his life negatively. The principle of preserving life therefore must rank above that of alleviating suffering.

Family preferences are irrelevant in this case, since his family abdicated all responsibility for him shortly after his birth. His institutional caregivers are legally bound to seek all possible treatment for him. The consequences to the institution of not treating him might be most unfortunate. These could include litigation, increased bureaucratic interference in the running of the institution, and the loss of what little discretionary power it now has. The harm inflicted on Arthur G. by ensuring his survival is surely outweighed by these long-range harms to the institution and its other residents, as well as by the harm which would be done to him were he to be deprived of life itself. For all these reasons, proceeding with the surgery seems to be not only medically indicated and legally required, but ethically appropriate as well.

With respect to the second case introduced at the beginning of this chapter, in my view the ethical obligation of the plastic surgeon to whom Sheila W. went initially for breast enlargement was to have refused to perform the silicone implantations. Hers was not a medical problem at all; if anything, it was psychological. This was certainly the nature of her husband's difficulties. Attitudinal rather than physical changes were indicated for them both.

It is a fact that the risks of this procedure far outweigh the benefits, which is why silicone implantations are illegal in most states.

The principle of nonmaleficence clearly applies in this case: the surgeon is obliged not to harm his patient. So does the principle of beneficence: it is the plastic surgeon's ethical duty to benefit his patient, not himself. For these reasons, it would have been more appropriate for the plastic surgeon to have referred the couple to a psychotherapist than to have performed the surgery. Of course, doing this would have cost him his fee. For the surgeon to have adopted this course, in turn, would have required considerable integrity, which is where an ethics of virtue could make a contribution. Unfortunately, the person to whom Sheila W. went with her problem did not demonstrate the qualities that we have come to expect of the "virtuous" physician.

4

The Squaring of the Trapezoid

A twenty-three-year-old man was found one night, stabbed through the heart, on a street in East Palo Alto. He was immediately rushed to the emergency department at Stanford University Hospital. From there he was taken into the operating room for heart surgery. The surgery was successful. The young man's heart was repaired. But after the operation he did not regain consciousness. Subsequent neurological tests revealed that he had sustained irreversible and almost total brain damage during the time he had lain bleeding on the street where he had been found. Instead of being pumped to his brain, his blood had flowed out into the gutter.

A month later, the physicians taking care of him came to the unanimous conclusion that this young man's life should no longer be sustained by artificial means and that he should be allowed to die naturally. The patient's father, who had lost his only other child in a drug-related violent incident seven months previously, refused to listen to any suggestion that his surviving son not now be treated as vigorously as possible. When told that the victim could lie in a vegetative state for the next forty years and would probably never again communicate meaningfully with anyone, his impassioned response was, "Even if I have to lead him around on a leash like a dog for the rest of his life, I want my boy alive, not dead." For several days, a stalemate ensued, with the father refusing all requests by the medical team to give them permission to stop treating the patient aggressively and to start caring for him palliatively. And then the problem was unexpectedly resolved when the young man went into cardiac arrest and died before he could be resuscitated.

Guiding Moral Principles

This tragic story illustrates a conflict between the four important moral principles identified in the last chapter as guiding the practice of medicine: *beneficence*, requiring the physician to do everything possible to preserve life; *nonmaleficence*, imposing on the physician the duty not to harm and to alleviate suffering; *autonomy*, which allows patients or their surrogates, in this case the boy's father, to be party to the decision-making process; and *justice, distributively understood*, which mandates the equitable allocation of our limited resources. In this case, the father's autonomy was opposed to all three of these other principles. Forty years ago such a conflict would not have arisen. It is essential that we try to understand why.

As we have seen, the Western tradition informing the practice of medicine, at least from the time the Hippocratic writings began to be collected, has been typically *deontological*. That is to say, medicine has adopted certain basic ethical principles as guides in approaching moral problems encountered in the course of the physician-patient relationship.

Until the mid-twentieth century, the practice of the physician was informed chiefly by just two primary moral principles: beneficence and nonmaleficence. Beneficence requires the physician to do everything possible to benefit the patient; above all, this requires the attempt to preserve the patient's life. Nonmaleficence imposes on the physician the duty not to harm the patient. As was mentioned earlier, it is summed up in the dictum, *primum non nocere*—above all, or first of all, do no harm. Where the benefits are uncertain or scant, the duty not to harm assumes more importance than the obligation to attempt heroically to help. A corollary of nonmaleficence is the duty to alleviate suffering. When life can no longer be preserved, alleviating the patient's suffering becomes the physician's first obligation.

Two other ethical principles, patient autonomy and justice, distributively understood, were, at best, secondary to the primary principles of beneficence and nonmaleficence and, at worst, overshadowed by them altogether. Right up until the middle of the twentieth century, the traditional relationship of the physician to these four principles might aptly be described as trapezoidal: As Figure 4-1 indicates, the physician was not equidistant from all four principles. Beneficence and nonmaleficence impinged immediately and directly on medical practice; autonomy and justice hardly at all.

Figure 4-1: Traditional Configuration of Basic Ethical Principles Impinging on the Physician

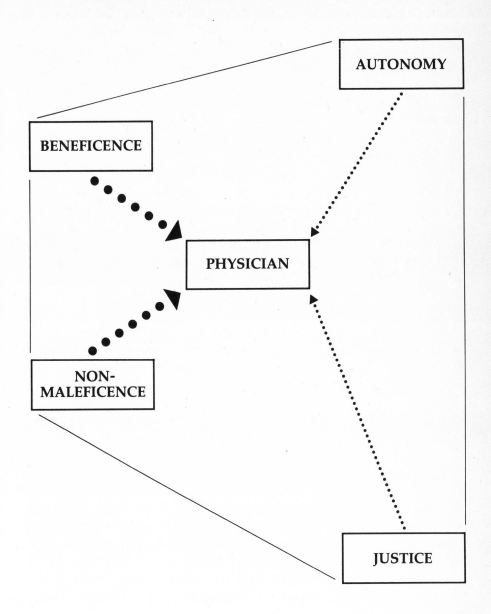

Autonomy

In the latter half of the twentieth century, the trapezoid underwent a metamorphosis and began to become a square. The process began with autonomy becoming the third primary ethical principle guiding the physician's practice in the United States. Autonomy requires that patients be regarded and respected as self-determining moral agents, as collaborators in attempting to restore health in the clinical setting or advancing the frontiers of medical knowledge, the goal of all medical research. Autonomy, which underlies the doctrine of informed consent, has come to command attention equal to that formerly given to the principles of beneficence and nonmaleficence for at least four discernible reasons.

First, there were the ghastly revelations of the Nuremberg trials, resulting in the Nuremberg Code of 1949 and the Helsinki Declaration of the World Medical Association of 1964. In these documents a reaction to the atrocities perpetrated by the Nazi doctors took the form of seeking to assure the autonomy of all subjects in research projects and requiring investigators to obtain from them voluntary and informed consents. Then, between 1963 and 1973 three cases came to light in the United States which further galvanized public opinion on the side of the consumer/subject.

The first was the Jewish Chronic Disease Hospital case (1963), in which three doctors, with approval from the director of medicine of the Jewish Chronic Disease Hospital in Brooklyn, New York, injected live cancer cells subcutaneously into twenty-two chronically ill and debilitated patients. Next, there was the case (1963) in which hepatitis was experimentally induced into mentally retarded children being admitted to the Willowbrook State School in New York. And then the Tuskeegee Syphilis Study came to public notice. Initiated with a group of black syphilitic males in 1932, this study was intended to examine the end-stage effects of the disease. Even after penicillin had been discovered as a cure for syphilis, the subjects were never informed that this drug was available. By the time the Tuskeegee experiment became common knowledge (1973), the subjects were either dead or demented.

These infamous cases gave impetus to the federal government's promulgation of guidelines in 1974 governing research with human subjects and setting standards for informed consent. The principle of autonomy underlies these guidelines.

Second, in the clinical setting, there were a number of significant court cases upholding patient autonomy. The first of these, the *Schloendorff* case, goes back to 1914. In this case Justice Cardozo issued a classic statement of the patient's right to self-determination:

> Every human being of adult years and sound mind has a right to determine what shall be done with his own body; and a surgeon who performs an operation without his patient's consent commits an assault, for which he is liable in damages.

No major advances in the doctrine of informed consent occurred in the next forty years. Then, between 1957 and 1971, what is called *battery theory* became more deeply entrenched.[1] At about the same time, the physician's duty to obtain an informed consent began to be grounded in liability rather than in battery;[2] that is to say, for a physician to perform any procedure without the patient's informed consent constitutes gross *negligence*, for which the physician may be liable in a court of law. Finally, the two streams converged into a unified doctrine of informed consent.[3] For our purposes, the point to be made is that all of these cases from 1957 onward refine our understanding of informed consent and entrench autonomy as a medico-moral principle as important as beneficence and nonmaleficence were and are.

Third, in the 1960s and 1970s the concerns of the consumer movement began to extend to health care. Building on the concepts of the eighteenth-century philosopher Immanuel Kant, who urged that human beings be regarded and treated as ends in themselves rather than as means to other ends, patients were encouraged to become autonomous, self-determining, assertive partners in relationships with physicians. The titles of several books written during this time make the point eloquently: *Managing Your Doctor; The Rights of Hospital Patients: The Basic American Civil Liberties Guide to a Hospital Patient's Rights; Talk Back to Your Doctor: How to Demand (and Recognize) High Quality Health Care; The Active Patient's Guide to Better Medical Care;* and *Our Bodies, Ourselves.*

And, finally, in the 1970s and early 1980s, several right-to-die initiatives and legislative measures further emphasized the principle of patient autonomy. The so-called Living Will, the Natural Death Act, the Durable Power of Attorney for Health Care, and then, in California, a new initiative (which failed to gain enough signatures to be placed on the ballot in November, 1988), A Humane and Dignified Death Act: A New Law Permitting Physician Aid-in-Dying, all attempt to extend patient autonomy either beyond the point of consciousness or competence, or into a new area, that of receiving physician assistance in having death actively hastened. By the mid-seventies, the trapezoid began to look something like Figure 4-2.

Justice

Then, in 1983, the first Diagnosis Related Group (DRG) system of reimbursement was introduced by the federal government. This meant that hospitals taking care of Medicare patients would be reimbursed only on the basis of average costs and no longer for actual expenditures. The era of seemingly unlimited resources, during which the use of high-cost, high-technology medical practices had been multiplying, was coming to an end. No longer could physicians, their patients, or their patients' insurers continue to ignore the expenses generated by defensive diagnostic tests and cavalier hospital admissions.

The urgent problem of the medically indigent, of whom there are now about 37 million, which had been concealed when hospitals could play the "Robin Hood Game"—taking from the rich to help the poor—became blatantly and scandalously obvious. Hospitals could no longer afford to provide free medical care to the indigent. They were required to send those patients who could not pay for services to designated county facilities, where long waits, overworked staff, and a generally lower quality of care were typical. The principle of distributive justice, which thrusts upon us the question, "How can we evenhandedly allocate our finite resources among the many who claim an equitable share?" could no longer be ignored. Finally, after 1983, the trapezoid became a square (Figure 4-3).

These late-twentieth-century historical, cultural, and economic phenomena have had a profound effect on the way in which moral principles impinge on the physician. The doctor now finds herself in the middle of a moral square, rather than inside the trapezoid which prevailed until the middle of the twentieth century. The four corners of the square—*beneficence, nonmaleficence, autonomy,* and *justice*—influence the physician equally. Those who practice medicine and provide medical services now must reckon with all four principles rather than with just the two primary guidelines of beneficence and non-

Figure 4-2: The Beginning of the Metamorphosis of the Trapezoid into a Square, after 1946

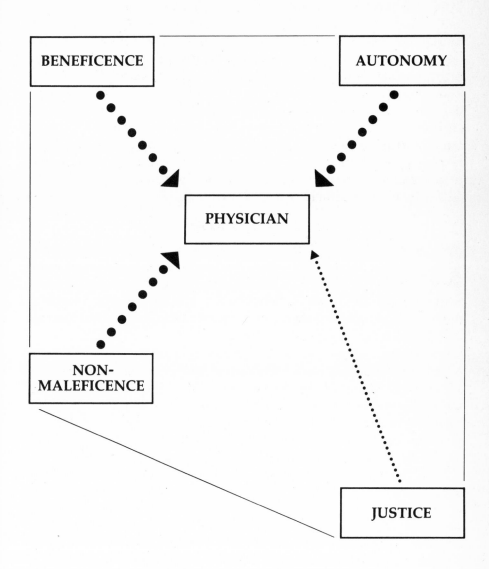

maleficence. The ramifications of this are far-reaching. We have not yet begun adequately to come to grips with them either in medical education or in postgraduate internship and residency training, or in the way we care for patients generally. These implications have made life infinitely more complicated for all who work in a medical care setting.

Each of the four principles mentioned is continually in tension—and potentially in conflict—with one or more of the others. The tension between beneficence and nonmaleficence is something with which we have long been familiar. These two primary medico-moral principles have always had to be balanced against each other. This is known as the risk-benefit ratio. Do the likely benefits of an intervention outweigh the possible risks attaching to it? Only if the answer is affirmative is it morally licit to proceed. And when patients such as our unfortunate stabbing victim can no longer be benefited by the heroic interventions of a modern intensive care unit, nonmaleficence requires that their suffering be alleviated and that these desperate means be either withheld or withdrawn.

Costs vs. Benefits

But in the latter half of the twentieth century we have to consider not only a risk-benefit calculus, but also the cost-benefit ratio. Are the costs of a particular diagnostic test or intervention warranted by the ensuing benefits? Or are the benefits marginal relative to the costs and therefore contraindicated? This need to evaluate is illustrated in another recent case.

The patient had been in the intensive care unit for several weeks. She had a lengthy previous medical history of chronic renal failure and diabetes. She was in the hospital because of a motor vehicle accident that resulted in several broken limbs and a possible head injury, as indicated by an altered mental status after the accident. Although often disoriented, she could follow simple commands.

Even after several weeks in the ICU, her physicians were unable to diagnose the source of her altered mental condition. Severe cerebral swelling was evident on a computerized tomographic (CT) scan, but nothing else. On the day before she was transferred from the ICU to the intermediate intensive care unit, the resident ordered another head CT scan, another electroencephalogram (EEG), a heart echogram, and a bone marrow biopsy. The nurses protested, not on cost-effective grounds, but for humanitarian reasons. The

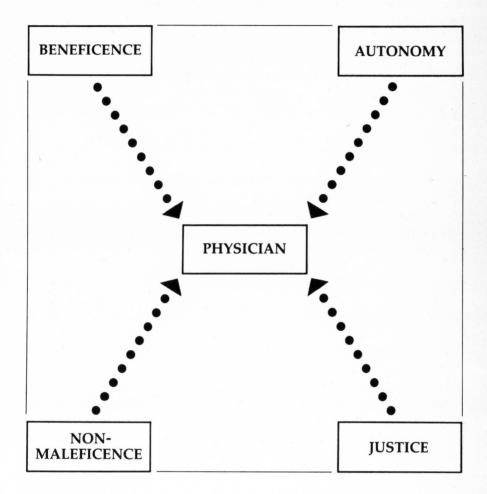

Figure 4-3: The Completion of the Metamorphosis of the Trapezoid into a Square, after 1983

attending physician, however, backed up the resident, and the tests—which produced no new diagnostic information—were done. The financial costs were enormous and unnecessary; the emotional cost borne by the patient was not even considered. Both the resident and the attending physician appear to have been oblivious to the requirements of the justice corner of the moral square.

It is perhaps in the area of intensive care, for the very young as well as for the very old, that cost-benefit considerations need most to be reckoned with. For the elderly, most medical expenditures accrue in the last year of life. Similarly, for an infant requiring neonatal intensive care, the first year of life is exorbitantly expensive. At both ends of life's spectrum, the question is inescapable: Would not our medical care dollars have a more telling effect if spent on relatively inexpensive rehabilitative or preventive medicine rather than on high-cost, high-technology, heroic interventions?

Not only are beneficence and justice in tension with each other; autonomy and justice can come into conflict as well. There is an inherent tension between what individuals want on the basis of autonomous choice and what society deems it fair to provide because of concerns about distributive justice.

This conflict became actual in the case with which we began—that of the twenty-three-year-old man found stabbed through the heart. Until it became certain that he had sustained massive and irreversible brain damage as a result of oxygen not being supplied to his brain, beneficence required that everything possible be done to save his life. Beyond that point, nonmaleficence as well as concerns about distributive justice made it reasonable to want to switch from aggressive to palliative care. But the young man's father, exercising autonomy as the patient's surrogate, continued to insist that everything possible be done for his son—even when this no longer made any sense either medically or economically. The wants of the individual were now at odds with the needs of society.

This case reminds us that no moral principle can or should ever be absolutized, which is why, in Figures 4-1, 4-2, and 4-3, the principles impinging on the physician are represented with dotted, rather than solid, lines. The father in this case wanted to absolutize autonomy and dictate medical care on the basis of his emotional need. The pro-life lobby would like to absolutize beneficence and save the life, for example, of every fetus no matter what the circumstances of the mother might be, and every neonate, however badly disabled and regardless of cost.

But principles have to be balanced against one another. Which is to assume priority over the others in any given situation must be decided rationally, by calculating the consequences of each of the options which are before us. This balancing is demanding, especially in the clinical setting, where time is of the essence and it is difficult to step back and think dispassionately about the implications of what is being attempted. But it is essential if we are to be responsive to all four principles that now comprise the moral square in which medicine must be practiced. This leads to three recommendations.

First, more research must be conducted on the cost-effectiveness, not only of new procedures and technologies, but also of those that have long been in place. As an example, in the sixties we had the resources, or thought we had, to pay $1,800 for each of the 2,500 hypothermia machines which were purchased and used in the United States to treat stomach ulcer patients with a procedure known as gastric freezing. Only after $4.5 million had been expended on these machines was the research done that established that gastric freezing not only was not helpful, but was actually harmful to patients, causing intestinal hemorrhaging! We can no longer afford such folly. Before new procedures and technologies are introduced and even after they have been adopted, their cost-effectiveness as well as their risk-benefit ratio needs to be evaluated. In light of this research, the practice of physicians must be modified, beginning in medical school, continuing through the house staff years, and on into private, group, or faculty practice programs.

Second, consumers have to be educated to understand that autonomy does not mean that we can have everything we want. In the philosophical literature, freedom has never been regarded as an absolute. It is always seen as the freedom of the individual consistent with the rights of others and one's responsibilities toward them. Autonomy is certainly not an absolute in the medical care setting. None of us has the right to command medical resources that are contraindicated both medically and in terms of fairness to others. Autonomy does not give us the license either to practice medicine, which is what the father of the young man who had been stabbed was actually attempting to do, or to make social policy on the basis of self-interest alone. Each of us is part of a community, and therefore the needs of the community have to be balanced against our own dreams and desires.

And, third, if we are to resolve the scandalous problem of America's 37 million medically indigent people, among the things all of us are going to have to accept is a reduction in the marginal benefits of medical care. This point is well made, for example, with reference to myocardial infarction.

Figure 4-4 shows schematically the aggregate net medical benefit of hospitalization for myocardial infarction plotted against the number of days of stay in the hospital. The first day of stay is typically the most beneficial. Each succeeding day offers less benefit, until a maximum is reached, here represented as occurring at day N. After that, some net harm might occur, taking into account the iatrogenic, that is, the hospital- or physician-induced, risks and the possible psychological harm of remaining in the hospital, represented by the slight downturn in the curve.

If the ideal period for treating myocardial infarction, assuming there were no complicating factors, was thought by a utilization review committee to be about 13 days, physicians at the far right of our diagram might be regarded as providing 5 days too much care. These 5 days would do the patient no net medical good and might do some

Figure 4-4: Aggregate Net Medical Benefit of Hospitalization*

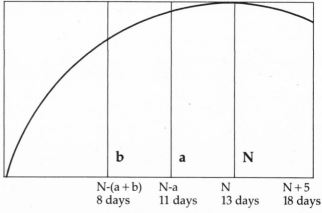

Days of Stay in Hospital

*Source: Robert M. Veatch, "DRGs and the Ethical Reallocation of Resources," *The Hastings Center Report*, vol. 16, no. 3, June 1986, pp. 32–40.

harm, thus violating both beneficence and nonmaleficence as moral guidelines. Similarly, autonomy might cause most of us to want 13 days of care, whereas considerations of distributive justice should compel us to see that if we accepted 11 days, or 8 days, the resources saved would not deprive us of more than marginal benefits and could at the same time benefit others, particularly the medically indigent. Getting all of us in society to settle for 11 days, or 8 days of hospital care will require a strenuous educational program leading to a radical shift in societal values.

In conclusion, consider another case history, which indicates that the four principles we have been considering can be balanced against one another in a way that makes sense for the patient, for the medical care providers, and for society's need to allocate its medical resources equitably.

The patient was a 43-year-old woman, with a history of chronic alcoholism. She was grossly obese and had sustained irreversible liver and kidney damage secondary to her alcoholism. She was brought into the hospital with a gastrointestinal hemorrhage. This required her to be transfused with two units of blood per day. All noninvasive attempts to locate the site of the hemorrhage were unsuccessful. Exploratory surgery was inadvisable because of her multiple medical problems. After a month she was on kidney dialysis, in liver failure, and still receiving two units of blood a day to sustain her life. There was no hope that any of her medical problems were reversible. Then she became febrile (feverish—indicating a possible infection). Her bedsores, secondary to her obesity, had become fistulae and, despite all efforts to heal them, had become infected. I was asked for an ethical consultation by the medical team. My recommendations and the outcome were as follows.

It was by now obvious that the principle of beneficence (mandating heroic attempts to preserve the patient's life) had to be subordinated to nonmaleficence (requiring the alleviation of her suffering) and distributive justice (calling for the conservation of scarce resources, not the least of which was the blood she was receiving) as the predominant guiding moral principles.

But the principle of patient autonomy had to be recognized as well. We did this by having an extended conversation with the patient in one of her completely lucid periods, when she was not being sedated for pain. In this session, she was provided with full information about her diagnosis, prognosis, and the various treatment options. It was suggested to her that the most appropriate decision from every possible point of view would be to stop treating her aggressively and to provide her with complete pain control so that she could have a peaceful and natural death. There were no relatives. We promised that she would not be alone when she died, that someone would be with her all the way. The patient concurred with these suggestions. Her infection was not treated. Her discomfort and pain were kept completely under control. Volunteers from the chaplaincy department stayed with her continuously, keeping vigil. Two days later, she succumbed to her infection. Hers was a truly good death.

5

Genetic Repair
and Enhancement

T he gene that causes fireflies to glow in the dark is wedded to the tobacco plant by means of recombinant DNA techniques, or "genetic engineering"; the tobacco plant becomes luminous by night. Patents are taken out on a novel, frost-resistant strawberry plant and a new strain of mouse, both developed using similar technology. A university committee criticizes one of its researchers, a plant pathologist, for injecting genetically altered bacteria into fourteen American elm trees in an experiment that apparently violates the university's research guidelines as well as those of the Environmental Protection Agency; the researcher terminates the experiment, in tears, by felling the elm trees with a chain saw.

A hormone produced through techniques of genetic manipulation is reported to raise the production of white blood cells in AIDS patients, thus helping them to ward off some infections. The genes of a sheep are introduced into those of a goat, and a "geep" is the result.

Hormones which once had to be harvested from fetal or infant cadaver tissue on a limited basis are now produced synthetically in specialized biochemical laboratories in unlimited quantities. Of such stuff are contemporary news headlines routinely made.

These developments signal the beginning of a genetic revolution, the end of which cannot even be imagined, let alone seen. Techniques for recombining deoxyribonucleic acid (DNA), the organic chemical of complex molecular structure occurring in cell nuclei as a constituent of chromosomes, where it serves to encode genetic data, have brought biomedical researchers and clinicians to the threshold of developing a high-resolution genetic map of the human organism, known as the *genome*, which would enable them to identify markers for some three thousand specific genetically linked diseases.

Inevitably, this in turn introduces the possibility of altering the genetic constitution of selected human patients, initially for therapeutic purposes and then, more sinisterly, by intervening directly in the evolutionary process itself so as to reconstitute the human species according to socially desirable qualities and characteristics. Ever since Adolf Hitler attempted by selective breeding to create a purely Aryan "master race," eugenic programs have been suspect in the civilized world. Genetic engineering could accomplish rapidly and exactly what selective breeding set out to achieve in markedly slower and less precise fashion.

The quandary faced by my friend, the biochemist whose research has brought him close to the point where he will have identified genetic markers for several devastating diseases—cystic fibrosis, certain types of breast cancer, schizophrenia, and possibly Alzheimer's—may, in fact, represent merely the moral tip of the genetic iceberg. Now that this work promises to be successfully completed, he worries about some of the possible consequences of the basic research he has been doing.

Ethical Problems

Leaving aside for now the issue of selective abortion where major genetic anomalies or abnormalities can already be identified (the diagnosis, for example, of Down's syndrome by means of amniocentesis), other major ethical problems associated with genetic diagnosis are likely to emerge soon. One is the old issue of truth-telling in new guise. What effect would there be on an otherwise healthy youngster of being told that in ten, twenty, thirty, or fifty years' time she will fall victim to a devastating disease—schizophrenia or Alzheimer's, for example? Would this information be beneficial or detrimental to the person concerned?

Another is the matter of confidentiality. In the absence of legislation prohibiting discrimination by insurers or employers on the basis of medical information demanded of applicants, those who are identified as having a genetic predisposition to serious diseases are clearly candidates for victimization. Even now, people with chronic diseases, such as diabetes or multiple sclerosis, or forms of cancer in remission have difficulty gaining employment and find it almost impossible to obtain health insurance. The confidentiality of one's medical record is no longer inviolate. Indeed, it is not an exaggeration to assert that in the computerized age in which we now live, strict confidentiality no longer exists.

Before genetic markers are identified for a whole range of devastating, late-onset diseases, steps need to be taken to provide legislative safeguards against discrimination on the basis of one's medical record. Those doing research in this area have a responsibility to be in the vanguard of the movement for the necessary legislative reform. Scientists cannot be indifferent to the moral consequences of their work. These are simply too serious and far-reaching.

Whether affected individuals ought to be informed beforehand about their potential medical problems and, if so, when, are tough questions. My belief that they should be told as soon as they are able to comprehend the significance of the information being imparted seems sound for two reasons. One is that truth-telling as a moral principle, coupled with appropriate emotional support, is preferable to paternalistic deception motivated by fear of the negative consequences of being honest. It expresses both respect for the personhood of the one being told the truth and a willingness to facilitate a constructive, rather than a destructive, response to it. Deception betrays a fundamental lack of respect for the humanity of others. It also excuses the deceiver from any need to continue to care for the emotional well-being of the recipient of grave news.

Another argument in favor of frankness is that once genetic markers for most serious diseases have been identified, the ability to diagnose may be expected to be followed soon thereafter by the capacity to treat. From diagnosis it will be but a short step to making available genetic therapies for conditions brought to light by means of genetic markers. Therefore, to withhold information about the diagnosis could deprive anyone identified as being predisposed to a devastating disease of an incipient treatment. This would be manifestly unfair. For both reasons, then, truth-telling seems indicated as a principle, always providing it is coupled with appropriate emotional support. This brings us to the central issues associated with genetic therapy to be addressed in this chapter.

Gene Therapy

With respect to the human species, the following two-by-two matrix[1] affords a convenient way of classifying the major categories of gene therapy now imminently available or on the horizon:

Somatic-cell repair	Germ-line repair
Somatic-cell enhancement	Germ-line enhancement

Somatic-cell repair has to do with the correction of a genetic defect in the somatic, or body, cells of an individual: solving the problem of diabetes, for example, not by means of insulin injections, but by replacing or repairing the gene which is failing to produce insulin in the cells of the pancreas.

Germ-line repair would involve the insertion of a functioning gene into the genetic makeup of a developing individual with a nonfunctioning gene; the disorder—failure to produce enough insulin, for example—would then be remedied, not only in the isolated cells of an affected individual, but also in his or her offspring.

Somatic-cell enhancement would entail the insertion of a gene into a genetically normal individual to try to improve or enhance a particular characteristic: placing an additional growth hormone gene into a normal child, for example, in order to produce an unusually tall basketball player or high jumper. The somatic-cell changes made would not be reproducible in offspring.

Germ-line enhancement, on the other hand, could be employed for eugenic purposes. The genetically altered characteristics of individuals could be transmitted, through sexual intercourse, to future generations. Hitler's fantasy of producing an "improved" version of the human species—more intelligent, taller, stronger, immune to the aging process, or whatever—could be attainable.

These four possibilities represent steps leading away from the morally and medically appropriate uses of genetic engineering to the inappropriate—from the acceptable to the unacceptable. Differentiating them from one another makes it clear why a simple answer is not possible to a question such as, "What is the moral propriety of genetic engineering?" Genetic engineering refers to disparate highly sophisticated biochemical techniques. The various uses to which these techniques may be put require close ethical scrutiny. With that in mind, we shall examine separately and on their own merits what we have called somatic-cell repair, germ-line repair, somatic-cell enhancement, and germ-line enhancement.

Somatic-cell Repair

The first procedure to be considered is the genetic repair of a single body cell. Plans have already been made to treat infants with three genetic diseases by this means.[2] In each case, the disease is caused by the absence of a single enzyme; all three are thus prime candidates for genetic enzyme repair.

- Lesch-Nyhan syndrome is a recessive condition linked to the X chromosome, involving a process of neurological and physiological deterioration from approximately the sixth month of life; the most striking feature of the syndrome is compulsive, uncontrollable self-mutilation.

- In adenosine deaminase deficiency (ADA,) the T and B lymphocytes are depleted, so that someone affected with the disease has no functioning immune system.

- Purine nucleoside phosphorylase deficiency (PNP) affects the B lymphocytes only, resulting in a selectively nonfunctioning immune system (which is why ADA is more swiftly lethal than PNP).

Because of the depletion of the B lymphocytes, and in the case of ADA, the T lymphocytes as well, children born with these diseases become vulnerable, within six months of birth, to the many virulent infections to which a compromised immune system is particularly prone. ADA deficiency usually results in death within a year of life;

a child with PNP would typically die within a few years. Both ADA and PNP may be likened to AIDS, the difference being that, as the name suggests, AIDS is an acquired immunodeficiency syndrome, whereas in ADA and PNP the immunodeficiency is innate.

Genetic therapy for these diseases would begin with the removal of some bone marrow. By means of a retroviral vector (retroviruses infect human cells and can therefore be used to transport DNA into cells), normal genes that will express the missing enzymes would next be inserted into the bone marrow. The treated bone marrow cells would then be reintroduced into the infant from whom they were taken. The expectation is that the treated cells will make good the deficiencies previously causing the respective diseases and that the infants treated will develop normally.

Three ethical criteria for experimental gene therapy, first proposed by W. French Anderson and John C. Fletcher in 1980,[3] serve as eminently sound moral guidelines. Prior to human clinical trials being undertaken, animal studies should demonstrate that

- New, curative genes can be directed to specific cells and remain there long enough to be effective (the criterion of delivery).

- The added genes will express their product in the target cells at a sufficient and appropriate level (the criterion of expression).

- No harm will result to the treated or surrounding cells, to the test animal, or to its offspring (the criterion of safety).

At this time, the only human tissue reliably available for gene transfer is bone marrow. Even in infants, bone marrow can be safely and successfully aspirated, grown in culture to allow for the introduction of exogenous "donor" genes, and then successfully reimplanted intravenously into the body of the infant from whom the tissue was taken. These techniques are well established and free of serious risk. It is simply not possible, given our present state of knowledge, to do the same thing with any precision via intravenous or intramuscular injection.

Even using bone marrow transfer, however, scientists are a long way from being able to use retroviruses as reliable vehicles for transporting the requisite DNA specifically to selected cells, let alone to much smaller predetermined chromosomal sites. This has been done in lower organisms, but such accuracy is not yet possible in mammals. From an ethical perspective, therefore, technical questions about effective delivery must be asked and answered satisfactorily in the animal model before the genetic repair of single body cells can be contemplated with human subjects.

Once an exogenous donor gene has been successfully delivered to the target cells of an organism, the next problem is to get it to function properly. Some success is beginning to be achieved with animal models, but there is a long way to go before transport mechanisms become available with all the regulatory signals necessary for the correctly controlled expression of exogenous genes in target cells in human beings. Until the criterion of expression is met satisfactorily in studies done with animals, it is premature to consider single-cell gene therapy in humans.

Safety is the third criterion. The exogenous retroviruses (remember, retroviruses infect human cells) used for gene transfer have several disadvantages. One is that they seem to be able to rearrange their own structure, as well as exchange sequences with other retroviruses; in other words, they are unstable. Thus, "there is the possibility that a retroviral vector might recombine with an endogenous viral sequence to produce an infectious recombinant virus."[4] It is even possible that such a virus could produce a malignant growth. Much work must be done *in vitro* ("in the glass," that is, in the laboratory) with bone marrow culture tissue, and then *in vivo* (with live organisms, usually first with mice and then with primates), to establish the safety of the delivery-expression system before it is used in humans. This appears to be the major obstacle yet to be overcome.

Once the three criteria of delivery, expression, and safety have been satisfied *in vitro* and *in vivo* with various mammals, including primates, Anderson argues that "it would [then] be unethical to delay human trials. . . . Arguments that genetic engineering might someday be misused do not justify the needless perpetuation of human suffering that would result from an unnecessary delay in the clinical application of this potentially powerful therapeutic procedure."[5]

This is a view with which I concur. The genetic repair of single cells is not categorically different from the surgical repair of single organs. In both cases, interventions are being attempted to correct either a nonfunctioning organ—kidney transplantation, for example—or a nonfunctioning enzyme. Once the standards of delivery, efficacy, and safety have been met, this form of treatment ought to be studied in clinical trials in humans, with a view to its eventually taking its place alongside currently established therapies such as surgery, radiation, or chemotherapy, alone or in combination. The principle of beneficence warrants a discrete advance along the lines suggested. If we can find a way to help infants who would otherwise die or live miserably survive intact to a healthy adulthood, the chance is worth taking. Single-cell gene therapy promises large benefits in treating several diseases for which at present there is no available remedy.

Germ-line Repair

Therapy for single cells, the effects of which will be transmitted into the affected individual's reproductive system, is the next possibility to be considered. Immediately, as we move from somatic-cell repair to germ-line repair, the stakes are raised. Treatments which would produce an inherited change, and could therefore pass on to future generations any negative traits inadvertently introduced into the germ-line, may have adverse consequences beyond our ability to foresee. To be able to repair genetic defects, not only in single cells, but in the germ line, so that the defect in question would no longer be passed on from one generation to the next, would demand extensive and major advances in our knowledge. The technical difficulties in the way of germ-line therapy are enormous. According to Anderson, "Germ line transmission and expression of inserted genes in mice has been obtained by several laboratories but with a technique that is not acceptable for use in human patients, namely, the microinjection of fertilized eggs."[6]

The technique is not acceptable for use with humans for the following reasons: (1) that the procedure has a high failure rate—the majority of eggs are so damaged by the microinjection and transfer procedures that they do not develop into live offspring; (2) that it can produce a deleterious result because there is no knowing where the injected DNA will be absorbed into the genome; (3) that it would have only limited usefulness in cases where both patients were homozygous for the defect, that is, where the defect would necessarily be expressed in their offspring, as distinct from heterozygous where the defect would be recessive. These technical difficulties would have to be overcome before there could be any thought of germ-line therapy in humans.

Even then, a major ethical concern, already alluded to, would remain. A treatment that produces an inheritable change, and could therefore perpetuate in future generations any mistake or unanticipated problems resulting from the therapy, is fraught with risk.[7] Even if it be argued that any negative traits inadvertently introduced into the germ line by means of genetic engineering could probably, by the same means, be later removed, this would only benefit those progeny who could be identified and located. Those not identified or located would be harmed, as would their offspring. The principle of nonmaleficence suggests that we should proceed along these lines with extreme caution.

Only when extensive experience has been accumulated with single-cell genetic therapy; only when animal studies have established that the criteria of delivery, expression, and safety can be met satisfactorily; and only after society has debated and consented to the taking of this serious next step, ought this kind of research with humans be allowed to proceed. Such research, of course, would be subject to the same moral and legal constraints governing all other kinds of research involving human subjects. And until clinical trials have been done, with statistically significant positive results, such investigative procedures ought never to be presented as therapy. With these qualifications, germ-line therapy might eventually be accepted as a logical next step following somatic-cell repair.

However, once we move from repair to enhancement, the issues become very different. Now we are no longer talking about the attempt to repair defective genes, either in single cells or in the germ line; we are thinking of enhancing or improving normal genes in ways dictated by the arbitrary tastes or aspirations of individuals. We are contemplating the possibility of making men of normal height even taller, women of normal proportions even bigger breasted, and gymnasts of normal strength and agility as strong and agile as chimpanzees. Considering the wide variety of devious means already used by Olympic athletes determined to enhance their performance—and Ben Johnson's fate attests to this—it is not stretching the imagination too far to envision genetic engineering being looked to for the attainment of similar ends.

Somatic-cell Enhancement

With respect to single-cell enhancement, we enter an area analogous to that now occupied by plastic surgeons who perform cosmetic, as distinct from reconstructive, procedures. Obviously, the techniques for genetic and surgical enhancement are quite different. However, there are both similarities and differences between them with respect to the ethical problems they raise.

Consider for a moment the moral implications of the plastic surgeon performing cosmetic procedures. Reconstructive procedures would include hand surgery to reconnect and restore function to an amputated finger or whole hand, facial skin grafts to restore beauty to someone disfigured by third-degree burns, and even sex-change operations when indicated for profound psychological and physiological reasons. For the most part, such procedures are morally uncontroversial. They are welcomed as beneficial contributions to the improvement of the human condition.

But cosmetic surgery is far more contentious. Making buttocks smaller, breasts larger, tummies flatter, faces less wrinkled, eyes less baggy, or noses shorter or straighter may be a legitimate business enterprise. But, *prima facie*, it belongs more in the domain of the beautician than of the physician. True, medically trained persons must perform these procedures. And, true, such surgeries often contribute extensively to the emotional and psychological well-being of those who undergo them. But they seem peripheral to the major purpose of medicine: to fight disease and to restore human beings to wholeness—so far as possible. Besides, they address psychological problems which may often be amenable to different approaches that are far less invasive and risky. As such, they do not necessarily express the ethical principles of beneficence and nonmaleficence.

Many types of cosmetic surgery are morally questionable for several reasons. One has already been alluded to. Even if there are emotional and psychological indications for performing cosmetic surgery, the procedures themselves seem more to ameliorate symptoms than to address underlying problems. Reflect, if you will, on the case of Sheila W., mentioned in the previous chapter. Her real problem was one of self-esteem. Until an attempt had been made to address that problem by the least invasive means available, namely, psychotherapy, it was unethical for the plastic surgeon to have performed a procedure as fraught with potential hazard as silicone breast implantations.

There may, indeed, be a place for cosmetic surgery as a treatment of last resort. But until less invasive means have been attempted for the alleviation of cosmetic problems—diet, exercise, and psychotherapy among them—to employ more invasive and potentially much more risky means such as cosmetic surgery seems self-serving and irresponsible. In sum, except as a treatment of last resort, cosmetic surgery appears to contradict the principles of beneficence and nonmaleficence.

Genetically engineered changes carry with them potentially greater risks than cosmetic surgical procedures—although the risks of stomach stapling as a treatment for obesity, for example, are not insignificant. There is no guarantee that attempting to provide a gymnast with the upper-body strength of a gorilla, for example, using recombinant DNA techniques to accomplish this, will not produce unforeseen adverse side effects—like increased hairiness on the hands, arms, and upper body or, more seriously, profound behavioral changes in the individual being "helped."

To move precipitously from repair to enhancement would be irresponsible. The justification for taking risks is greater when the attempt is being made to remedy a defect not amenable to correction by other, less dangerous, means than it is when one is merely wanting to improve on nature. The financial cost of doing genetic enhancement would also be higher than the cost, say, of cosmetic surgery. At the moment, the expense of research is being met largely with federal research grants. To apply the techniques that will eventually flow from such research to enhance the normal attributes of an elite group within our society, i.e., those who can afford to pay for it, represents a misuse of public funds. Surely, we have more urgent national medical priorities.

Nevertheless, there is one category of enhancement genetic engineering which may be ethical: that which falls under the rubric of preventive medicine. An example would be treatment for atherosclerosis (hardening and clogging of the arteries)—a major cause of strokes and heart attacks. The incidence of these maladies is correlated with cholesterol levels in the blood. If it were established that an increased number of low density lipoprotein (LDL) receptors on body cells would result in lower blood cholesterol levels, then "the insertion of an additional LDL receptor gene in 'normal' individuals could significantly decrease the morbidity and mortality caused by atherosclerosis."[8]

However, now that several new pharmacological means of accomplishing this have been developed, approved by the FDA, and are in common use, one wonders whether the argument for doing the same thing genetically has as much force. The principle on which this concern rests is that of nonmaleficence. In order to do as little harm as possible, a more invasive and riskier procedure ought never to be used when a less invasive and less risky alternative is available. Only markedly superior benefits can justify the exposure of the person being treated to dangers greater than those associated with already available conventional therapies.

Germ-line Enhancement

Here we enter the realm of eugenic genetic engineering— intervening directly in the evolutionary process in order to reconstitute human beings according to selected social criteria in ways that will be reproducible across the generations. The notion of creating a "super race," whether à la William Shockley, with his sperm bank "for geniuses only," or according to the ideology of an Adolf Hitler, is generally abhorrent in the Western world. The philosophical and theological conundrum of what constitutes the *humanum*—of what makes us quintessentially human beings—has not yet been unraveled with enough societal unanimity for us even to approach agreement on what the goals of eugenic genetic engineering should be.

An earlier book in the Portable Stanford series by Philip H. Rhinelander reminds us that we humans are still largely incomprehensible to ourselves.[9] The various views of human nature propounded by Plato, Marx, Freud, B.F. Skinner, and other major thinkers are essentially incompatible.[10] If the attempt were made to use genetic means to reconstitute our human nature in the germ line, which of these disparate visions would inspire the blueprints? And why? And what about those whose understanding of what it is to be human differs from that of the proponents of the predominant ideology?

Eugenics may be possible only within a totalitarian society. In a society as pluralistic as our own, as proud of its tolerance of diversity as ours is, and as jealous of its freedoms, the very thought of molding human nature to fit societally determined ends is repulsive. Even if it were technically possible to think of germ-line enhancement, our moral and philosophical resistance to it would be too vigorous for it to succeed. The struggle for civil rights for minorities in this country has been too hard and has taken too long for these precious gains to be squandered lightly on any decision that human beings of only a certain kind ought to be perpetuated. As one leading commentator puts it:

> At face value, the attainment of eugenic aims conflicts strongly with liberty. The implementation of eugenic programs has historically entailed selective, and often arbitrary and coercive, restrictions on some members of society and not others. The problem of justice is exacerbated by the fact that by definition the negative aspects of any eugenic policy on liberties would be directed at the least, rather than the most, fortunate members of society.[11]

In conclusion, once the criteria for ethical research detailed earlier have been met, there is no reason to object on moral grounds to the attempt to repair defective body cells in human beings by means of genetic engineering. Indeed, genetic engineering might supply valuable new weapons to the armamentarium of modern medicine for use in its fight against disease. If this proves to be the case, the principle of beneficence would require their adoption.

The technical and moral stakes are raised when we move from single-cell to germ-line therapy. There is, however, no inherent moral objection to this possibility. Ensuring delivery, expression, and safety will be more difficult than in single-cell therapy. Here, the principle of nonmaleficence is our primary guide. However, once these obstacles have been overcome to the satisfaction of experts in the field, the principle of beneficence would again sanction clinical trials in humans involving germ-line therapy.

Genetic enhancement, on the other hand, has disturbing implications. These are serious enough with respect to single-cell enhancement on the basis of the principle of nonmaleficence. They become positively alarming when germ-line enhancement is considered, not only because the risks are likely to outweigh the benefits, but because of the sociopolitical implications of justice. Some human beings would be used merely as means to others' eugenic ends in violation of the principle of respect for persons. It is here, therefore, that there is an urgent and imperious need for public debate. For only as we make up our minds as a society about these possibilities beforehand will we be able to prevent the abuse of our dawning technological expertise in this area.

Fortunately, the state of the art of genetic engineering is still relatively primitive. Leading researchers at Stanford, for example, are still working with bacteria, plants, and mice. There is, at present, no thought whatever of experimenting with primates, let alone human beings. A decade from now, the only work that will possibly be done with human beings will be at the single-cell level. This allows us breathing space—and hope. For here we may have an example of one of the few fields in modern scientific endeavor where possibilities outstrip accomplishments. There is yet time to consider the implications of what we will soon be able to achieve. This makes it imperative that we consider placing off limits some of the ends in the service of which the techniques of genetic engineering might eventually be employed. Our freedom carries with it a sometimes heavy but necessary burden of responsibility.

6

The New Reproductive Technologies

Bill, 42 years of age, and Barbara, 39, are both professionals. They have been married for seven years. This is Bill's first marriage, Barbara's second. She has two children, now teenagers, from her previous marriage. Although their marriage has been at times tempestuous, in part because Bill has had to establish intimate working relationships with three people, not merely one, Bill and Barbara care deeply about each other. Having reached a position, financially, to consummate their union by having a child of their own, they assiduously attempted this—without success. Barbara knew that she was fertile; she had two children to prove it. It seemed that the problem of infertility was Bill's. He underwent tests, then surgery to improve his sperm count, but to no avail. Then Barbara consulted a fertility specialist and had a gynecological examination. This revealed some endometriosis—inflammation and then scarring of the uterine tissue. Barbara, too, had surgery to correct this problem. Still, their infertility persisted.

The fertility specialist then suggested in vitro *fertilization—extracting several of Barbara's ova (eggs), mixing them with Bill's sperm in a petri dish, and then reimplanting one or more of the fertilized eggs into her uterus at the appropriate time. Each attempt cost between $5,000 and $6,000. Bill and Barbara tried in vitro *fertilization on two separate occasions— again to no avail. Desperate for a child, they now contemplated Barbara's having artificial insemination with donor sperm. Bill's best friend was willing to donate his sperm; Bill was happy for him to do so. Barbara demurred.

Before giving up on the dream she and Bill shared of having a child of their own, she wanted them to attempt a procedure of last resort: Bill wearing a testicular cooling device for several months in the hope of improving his *sperm count. Bill agreed to do this despite the obvious inconvenience (not to say embarrassment) involved. Finally, less than a year later, this strategy proved successful. Barbara became pregnant by Bill.*

Infertile couples privately bear a poignant burden. It has been estimated that there are almost three million couples in the United States wanting to have children of their own yet unable to do so. The sadness occasioned by the denial of their wish to have babies must surely be intensified both by the fertility of friends and by the shortage of normal, healthy infants available for adoption.

The difficulty is pervasive. In part, it represents a dark facet of the women's revolution. As more and more women are enjoying independent professional careers outside the home, childbearing and childrearing are being deferred. Yet women appear to be at the peak of their reproductive powers in their late teens and twenties; it is in their late thirties and early forties that many women who have delayed having children become acutely aware of the ticking of their biological clocks. Before it is too late to have children or too risky, both for the mother and for the baby, the reproductive urge asserts itself. All too frequently impediments to fertility then emerge.

These problems are complex. They manifest themselves, physiologically speaking, either in the male or the female partner, or in both, and are surely compounded by the emotions typically evoked by infertility: anxiety, tension, jealousy, resentment, and fear. Until recently, not much could be done except to offer artificial insemination to the female partner, with the sperm either of the husband or of a donor. This expedient was unhelpful where the difficulty stemmed from the woman's own inability to ovulate or conceive or, if conception did occur, from the failure of the conceptus to implant in her uterus.

Then, in July 1978, the birth occurred of the first child in human history who was the product of *in vitro* fertilization—the uniting of sperm and ova in the laboratory, with fertilized eggs being implanted into the woman's womb. As the *Warnock Report* described it, "The technique, long sought, at last successful, opened up new horizons in the alleviation of infertility and in the science of embryology."[1] Since that time, thousands of similar births have occurred around the globe. A new subspeciality of obstetrics-gynecology has come to be recognized: that of the fertility specialist. And a variety of sophisticated pharmacological and surgical means of combating problems of infertility have been devised.

Several alternatives to natural procreation have now been developed. At least sixteen discrete possibilities warrant a brief mention:

- Artificial insemination of the wife by her husband

- Artificial insemination of the wife by a donor

In the following four instances, fertilization occurs in the laboratory, the embryo is implanted into the *wife's* uterus, and she carries the resulting baby to term:

- *In vitro* fertilization of the wife's ova with the husband's sperm

- *In vitro* fertilization of the wife's ova with donor sperm

- *In vitro* fertilization of a donor's ova with the husband's sperm

- *In vitro* fertilization of a donor's ova with a donor's sperm

In the next two, fertilization occurs in the uterus of a second woman from whose uterus the embryo is lavaged (washed out), to be implanted into the *wife's* uterus:

- Artificial insemination with the husband's sperm of a woman other than the wife

- Artificial insemination with a donor's sperm of a woman other than the wife

In the following two instances, fertilization occurs in the wife; the embryo is lavaged from her uterus and is implanted into that of a *surrogate*, who carries the baby to term:

- The wife is impregnated with her husband's sperm

- The wife is impregnated with a donor's sperm

In the following six examples, fertilization occurs in the laboratory, with the embryo being implanted into the uterus of a *surrogate*, who carries the baby to term:

- *In vitro* fertilization of the wife's ova with the husband's sperm

- *In vitro* fertilization of the wife's ova with a donor's sperm

- *In vitro* fertilization of a donor's ova with the husband's sperm

- *In vitro* fertilization of a donor's ova with donor sperm

- *In vitro* fertilization of a surrogate's ova with the husband's sperm

- *In vitro* fertilization of a surrogate's ova with donor sperm—what might be called "planned procreation for placement."

The first two represent the alternative to childlessness traditionally available: artificial insemination by husband or by donor. It is estimated that more than 10,000 conceptions occur annually in the United States through artificial insemination. Perhaps the single major ethical concern about artificial insemination is its relationship to marriage and the consequences it has for the meaning of parenthood.[2]

Ethical Issues

The next four categories all represent variations on the theme of *in vitro* fertilization (IVF). Three major ethical concerns about *in vitro* fertilization have to do with the use of "spare" embryos, the "culling" of multiple pregnancies, and the resource allocation issue raised by the cost of this procedure. A further brief elaboration of these three concerns is warranted.

In order to maximize the possibility of a successful birth resulting from IVF at the first try, more ova are fertilized than are strictly necessary. Of these, only one or two may be implanted into the wife's uterus, leaving "spare" fertilized ova (embryos) to be frozen and stored for future use should the first attempt at IVF and implantation be unsuccessful. Alternatively, all of the embryos may be implanted and, later, if a multiple pregnancy ensues, several of the resulting fetuses may be aborted ("culled") to leave the couple with one or two viable children, at most, rather than five or six whose chances of survival may be minimal.

Both practices are morally problematic. With respect to the first, the cryopreservation (freezing) of embryos, one celebrated case involved a husband and a wife who were both killed in an airplane accident, leaving behind them two "spare" frozen embryos, resulting from their own ova and sperm, the husband's son from a previous marriage, now in his mid-twenties, and a considerable estate. Not the least of the legal and moral quandaries presented by this case were the questions of what was to be done with the frozen embryos and what was their status regarding inheritance before the law.

Other ethical questions associated with cryopreservation persist as well: does the freezing and thawing of embryos result in abnormal or defective births? (No evidence thus far suggests that it does.) Does the embryo itself have rights before implantation? Is the freezing of embryos an acceptable intrusion into the natural process of reproduction?

The second approach, in which all of the available embryos are implanted, is equally contentious. The human reproductive system is notably inefficient: of one hundred eggs exposed to potential fertilization among fertile couples, only thirty-one will produce viable offspring. Hence, multiple embryo transfer promises a higher success rate than the transfer of single embryos—and is likely to be less costly than repeated procedures each involving a single embryo. This means that if the initial procedure succeeds, the result could be a multiple pregnancy, anything from quintuplets to octuplets.

The larger the number of babies a woman is carrying, the less likelihood there is that any of them will survive. Hence the need selectively to abort some of the fetuses to make it possible for those who remain to develop normally. Which should be sacrificed? And is it morally acceptable to sacrifice *any* for the sake of the one or two who will go on to become full-term babies? Does not this practice erode the notion that human beings are ends in themselves, and ought never to be treated as means to other ends?

The third moral issue presented by *in vitro* fertilization has to do with the allocation of scarce resources and the principle of justice, distributively understood. As was mentioned earlier, the cost of *in vitro* fertilization per treatment cycle is approximately $5,000 to $6,000; the success rate is about 15 percent. This means that the cost of a baby produced by this means would average at least $33,000 to $39,000.[3] Since *in vitro* fertilization results in a higher than usual number of premature births, it is probable that additional substantial costs associated with neonatal intensive care would be incurred—anything from $38,000 to $500,000.

One disquieting conclusion to be drawn from this is that this new technology, like so many others, would be available only to those with the financial means to pay for it and unavailable to those without. It raises a further searching question about health care priorities in an era of shrinking resources on the one hand and global overpopulation on the other. In light of other urgent, unmet needs and the worldwide population explosion, is this really something we should be doing, no matter how intensely couples may want to have children of their own? I am not convinced that we should.

Surrogate Motherhood

Artificial insemination is combined with what has come to be known as embryo transfer. In the first example, a surrogate for the wife is artificially inseminated with the husband's sperm. At an appropriate developmental moment, the resulting conceptus/embryo is washed (lavaged) out of the surrogate's uterus and is transferred to the uterus of the wife, who then carries the baby, it is to be hoped, to term. In the next example, a surrogate for the wife is artificially inseminated with sperm from a donor, a surrogate for the husband. The resulting embryo is subsequently transferred to the uterus of the wife, who then carries the baby—again, if all goes well, to term. Obviously, this is a more complicated and difficult procedure. The risks of failure and of success, since two surrogates are involved, increase concomitantly.

The final eight procedures are all different forms of what has come to be known as surrogate motherhood. That is to say, in each of them, the baby will be carried by a surrogate for the mother who, by agreement, is expected to hand the child over to the contracting couple after the birth has occurred.

In addition to raising serious questions about responsible resource allocation, these therapies involving *in vitro* fertilization present at least two further moral problems. One is the difficulty of what is to be done with "spare" embryos, those frozen and kept in storage. To whom do these belong? To the couple? What if the couple is divorced before the embryos can be implanted? Will custody battles of the future extend into the laboratory? Or do these embryos belong to the fertility specialist, to be used to help other infertile couples or for research, or to be flushed down the drain? These questions veil a prior unresolved, possibly unresolvable, perplexity: is an embryo to be regarded as human, or potentially human, or as merely a conglomeration of cells? This concern underlies the abortion debate as well.

The second issue raised by *in vitro* fertilization is that of the "culling" of multiple pregnancies—the current euphemism for this form of abortion. For those who believe in the potential, if not the actual, personhood of fetuses, this presents a profound ethical stumbling block.

The final two options differ from the preceding six in that they do not require *in vitro* fertilization and embryo transfer and implantation. In the next to last, of which "Baby M" is the most celebrated example, the husband's sperm is artificially inseminated into the surrogate mother, who bears the resulting child and then, if all works out as originally planned, hands the baby over to the contracting couple. In the last, something similar would happen, only with sperm from a donor rather than from the husband. In both cases, the surrogate mother is also the biological parent of the resulting child; the other biological parent is either the contracting father or the man donating the sperm.

Compounding the technical difficulties of these procedures are the financial transactions that occur between the contracting parties and those who arrange them, as well as moral and legal issues of the most vexed and far-reaching sort. These perplexities are clearly focused for us in the recent case of Baby M. It will be convenient, therefore, to discuss the moral issues associated with this arrangement and procedure alone.

The Case of Baby M

The case of Baby M, as is well known, involves two couples, the Stearns and the Whiteheads. The Stearns wanted children, but it seemed risky for Mrs. Stearn to conceive and bear a child of her own because she had symptoms of multiple sclerosis, a disease which could be aggravated by pregnancy. So the Stearns contracted with Mrs. Whitehead to bear a child for them. She would be artificially inseminated with Mr. Stearn's sperm. She would conceive and bear a child. And she would hand the child over to the Stearns for the sum of $10,000. Not often mentioned with respect to this case is the fact that those who arranged the transaction between the Stearns and the Whiteheads also received the sum of $10,000 for their "labor." The only difference was that they received their $10,000 beforehand. Mrs. Whitehead was to receive reimbursement only upon delivery of the child.

The story did not unfold according to plan. After giving birth to her baby, Mrs. Whitehead declined the $10,000 due to her and attempted to keep the child. She claimed, quite rightly, that it was her baby as much as it was Mr. Stearn's. The case went to court, and on March 31, 1987, the verdict went in favor of the Stearns—not without several gratuitous references to Mrs. Whitehead's fitness to mother the child she had borne. Her visitation rights were stripped from her. Then, on March 3, 1988, the New Jersey Supreme Court overturned that decision and granted to Mrs. Whitehead the visitation rights that are normally accorded biological parents who later divorce. It also banned the type of commercial surrogate contracts that had led to Baby M's conception by artificial insemination.

The legalities of this case are outside my sphere of competence.[4] My concern is with matters suggested by ethical reflection on the protracted saga of Baby M. The morality of surrogate motherhood has been widely debated. Well-defined opposing viewpoints have begun to emerge.

Religious, Ethical, and Legal Positions

The most unequivocal and uncompromising of these is the official stance of the Vatican. The Congregation for the Doctrine of the Faith has instructed Roman Catholics not to avail themselves of any non-natural means of procreation. This position is internally consistent with the Roman Catholic Church's teaching on sexuality, procreation, contraception, and abortion. Just as sex without the intent to make babies was previously frowned upon, so now making babies without sex is condemned:

> The origin of a human person is the result of an act of giving. The one conceived must be the fruit of his parents' love. He cannot be desired or conceived as the product of an intervention of medical or biological techniques; that would be equivalent to reducing him to an object of scientific technology.[5]

Most non-Roman Catholics and many Americans who are Roman Catholics find this doctrine unpersuasive and curiously out of touch with the needs and aspirations of people living in the modern world.

The *Warnock Report* was produced in Britain by the first national commission appointed to explore the ethical and legal implications of the new reproductive technologies. Its members included Dame Mary Warnock, a distinguished philosopher, as chairperson; a prominent theologian; several eminent legal counsels; various celebrated physicians representing the disciplines of obstetrics and gynecology, neurology, family medicine, and embryology as well as social workers, psychologists, and a health service administrator. The committee acknowledged that "the question of surrogacy presented us with some of the most difficult problems we encountered."[6] Nevertheless, it reached the following forthright conclusion, less reactionary than that of the Vatican, but still largely restrictive:

> We recommend that legislation be introduced to render *criminal* the creation or the operation in the United Kingdom of agencies whose purposes include the recruitment of women for surrogate pregnancy or making arrangements for individuals or couples who wish to utilize the services of a carrying mother; such legislation should be wide enough to include both profit and non-profitmaking organizations. We further recommend that the legislation be sufficiently wide to render criminally liable the actions of professionals and others who knowingly assist in the establishment of a surrogate pregnancy.
>
> We do not envisage that this legislation would render private persons entering into surrogacy arrangements liable to criminal prosecution, as we are anxious to avoid children being born to mothers subject to the taint of criminality. We nonetheless recognize that there will continue to be privately arranged surrogacy agreements. While we consider that most, if not all, surrogacy arrangements would be legally unenforceable in any of their terms, we feel that the position should be put beyond any possible doubt in law. *We recommend that it be provided by statute that all surrogacy agreements are illegal contracts and therefore unenforceable in the courts.*[7]

In Australia, a law prohibiting all commercial forms of surrogate motherhood was established following recommendations by a committee under the direction of Louis Waller, a law professor.[8]

A little more than two years later, the Ethics Committee of the American Fertility Society issued its report, *Ethical Considerations of the New Reproductive Technologies.*[9] The committee had reservations about surrogate motherhood, which focused on "the potential effects on the surrogate, the couple, the potential child, and society."[10] Its recommendations were somewhat less restrictive than those of the Warnock and Waller committees:

> The Committee believes that there are not adequate reasons to recommend legal prohibition of surrogate motherhood, but the Committee has serious ethical reservations about surrogacy that cannot be fully resolved until appropriate data are available for assessment of the risks and possible benefits of this alternative.
>
> The Committee recommends that if surrogate motherhood is pursued, *it should be pursued as a clinical experiment. Among the issues to be addressed in the research on surrogate mothers are the following:*
>
> a) the psychological effects of the procedure on the surrogates, the couples, and the resulting children
>
> b) the effects, if any, of bonding between the surrogate and the fetus *in utero*
>
> c) the appropriate screening of the surrogate and the man who provides the sperm
>
> d) the likelihood that the surrogate will exercise appropriate care during the pregnancy
>
> e) the effects of having the couple and the surrogate meet or not meet
>
> f) the effects on the surrogate's own family of her participation in the process
>
> g) the effects of disclosing or not disclosing the use of a surrogate mother or her identity to the child
>
> h) other issues that shed light on the effects of surrogacy on the welfare of the various persons involved and on society.[11]

My own position lies closer to the liberal side of the spectrum of opinions we have reviewed than to the restrictive end. Generally speaking, I favor surrogacy arrangements, but with three major reservations. These have to do with issues of *convenience, commercialization,* and *consent.*

Convenience

Where there is a genuine medical history of infertility or medical indications that pregnancy would be detrimental or even hazardous to a woman's health, it seems to me that she should not be prevented from having children with the help of a surrogate. However, the prospect of women resorting to surrogates, not because of medical indications, but for reasons of convenience, is alarming.

In a former era, fashionable and wealthy women, concerned that breast-feeding their infants would have a deleterious effect on their figures, hired wet nurses to do their nursing for them. Invariably, wet nurses were drawn from a lower social stratum, where there was a pressing financial incentive to engage in this once common occupation and where concerns about the loss of a tight bustline were ranked far lower on the scale of operative values. It is conceivable that wealthy, fashionable, career-minded women today would similarly be inclined to hire other women to bear their children for them. If nursing a baby is detrimental to one's figure, pregnancy and confinement can be much more so. Yet the risks associated with breast-feeding are infinitesimal compared with those of childbearing. The Warnock Committee commented on this particular point:

> We are all agreed that surrogacy *for convenience alone,* that is, where a woman is physically capable of bearing a child but does not wish to undergo pregnancy, is totally ethically unacceptable. Even in compelling medical circumstances the danger of exploitation of one human being by another appears to the majority of us to far outweigh the potential benefits, in almost every case. That people should treat others as a means to their own ends, however desirable the consequences, must always be liable to moral objection.[12]

A caveat is in order at this juncture. There will be times when it will be difficult in the extreme to draw a clear line between "compelling medical circumstances" and convenience. Mrs. Stearn, in the Baby M story, is a case in point. During the court hearing, evidence was brought forward to support the argument that she was not medically infertile but had symptoms of a disease (multiple sclerosis) which pregnancy would exacerbate. Having read carefully every report of the trial I could lay hands on, I found myself still uncertain about whether the motive for the contract with Mrs. Whitehead was convenience or not. Obviously, the physician involved in a surrogacy arrangement will be in the best position to make this judgment, but it will not always be obvious or unequivocal. The motives of human beings are notoriously difficult to discern, even when we are looking into our own hearts, let alone those of others!

Commercialization

Turning again to the facts of the Baby M case, it boggles the mind that the legal intermediaries who arranged the contract between the Stearns and the Whiteheads received as much money as Mrs. Whitehead herself. Further, as we have seen, they received their remuneration ahead of time, while she was offered payment only after Baby M's birth. This concentrates attention on the powerful financial incentive there is to commercialize surrogate motherhood.[13]

The members of the Warnock Committee in Britain had good reason to be exercised about the commercialization of surrogacy. At the time they were deliberating, I was on sabbatical in England, at Green College, Oxford University. The rate of unemployment in Britain then stood at 14 percent; the bulk of the unemployed were young men and women. Appearing daily in the London newspapers were classified advertisements, placed by Americans, offering $30,000 to British women who were willing to serve as surrogate mothers for them. To young, unemployed working-class women, $30,000 was undoubtedly an enormously large sum of money. Most of them would have been willing to do almost anything for such an inducement. It seemed to me then, as it does now, that when to convenience is added commercialization, the prospects for exploitation increase exponentially.

A rejection of the commercialization of surrogacy should not preclude fair remuneration to the surrogate for her expenses and time. But such compensation could be afforded without resort to financially motivated intermediaries. Just as many of our finest medical centers and hospitals are nonprofit institutions, it seems possible to sanction not-for-profit clinics where surrogacy agreements could be worked out in a way that would be fair to all parties concerned and exploitative of none. On this point I take issue with the Warnock

Committee, which recommended that not-for-profit as well as for-profit surrogacy organizations be rendered criminal.

It is arguable that there is no such quality as pure altruism. Even the best of human behaviors appear to be motivated by the desire to be rewarded—in nontangible as well as tangible ways. However, many of the reports of fertile women who have been willing to act as surrogate mothers for their infertile sisters or friends suggest that their motivation was largely altruistic. These stories are moving in the extreme. They inspire the belief that there is still alive in our culture a willingness to serve and to sacrifice for others. The commercialization of surrogacy is inimical to that spirit.

Consent

In entering into a surrogacy agreement with the Stearns, Mrs. Whitehead assented intellectually to an arrangement which, nine months later, she found it impossible to conclude because of the unexpected and powerful emotions evoked by her bonding with Baby M during the pregnancy. This raises concerns about the whole process of informed consent in acute and poignant fashion.

How can a woman possibly understand ahead of time what she will feel nine months later when, after carrying a baby to term and bonding with her, the day comes to part with her irrevocably and hand her over to someone else? The emotions she will likely experience can be described to her beforehand. She may think and believe that she will be able to deal with them positively. But the reality may turn out to be very different from what had been anticipated. Quite unexpectedly, her heart may prompt her to dissent from an agreement to which she had previously assented intellectually. Clearly, this happened to Mrs. Whitehead.

This one difficulty alone causes me to believe that prior to any surrogacy contract being entered into, the surrogate mother—and her husband, if she is married—should be required to undergo extensive psychological counseling. Means should be devised, not merely to describe to her ahead of time what emotions she is likely to feel when the moment comes to honor her agreement, but also to enable her actually to experience these anticipated feelings. In other words, substantial understanding of what she is committing herself to should be striven for in emotional as well as intellectual terms. Only after those providing her with counseling are satisfied that she will, indeed, be able to deal positively with the powerful feelings generated by parting with a child she herself has carried and delivered should she be allowed to enter into the surrogate contract. This may take weeks of patient work, if not months.

The difference between fair compensation for services rendered and the offer of an irresistibly high inducement—the $30,000 held out to young British women who were willing to become surrogates for American mothers in the example previously cited—might mean the difference between a substantially voluntary and a manipulated or even coerced decision, according to how poor the woman volunteering is.

Commercialized surrogacy is bound to appeal less to altruism than to materialism as a motivating force. Such motivation may prove inadequate when it comes to dealing with the emotions subsequently triggered when the baby is to be handed over to the party or parties contracting for the services of the surrogate mother. This leads to a paradoxical conclusion, based on surmise rather than proof: as a motive for entering into a surrogacy contract, altruism, rather than materialism, would appear to hold out a better promise of achieving the desired results—to the satisfaction of all parties concerned.

Implicit in the whole notion of an informed consent is the authentic possibility of an informed refusal. With some exceptions, such as agreement to surgical procedures, consent is usually revocable. It may later be withdrawn, and the agreed upon procedures or studies may be refused. The right to refuse treatments previously consented to is now well recognized: by the American Medical Association, the American Hospital Association, and in case law. Even in the research setting. most informed consent forms include a paragraph that affords the subject the right to withdraw from the study, for any reason, at any time.

However, consent to a legally binding contract is not usually or easily revocable. The challenge surrogate motherhood presents to morality and the law is how to allow for an informed refusal and at the same time to ensure that the contract will be binding. One way of meeting this difficulty might be to allow a grace period of, say, six weeks after the birth of the child, during which time the surrogate could change her mind and decide to keep the baby rather than give it away—with appropriate penalties, including forfeiture of the agreed upon compensation for services rendered. This would be similar to the six-month period allowed to a mother who offers her child for adoption. During these six months she is free to change her mind.

Once the six months have elapsed she is not, and the adoption contract becomes legally binding.

Admittedly, this would place a severe burden of anxiety on the couple contracting with a surrogate. For six weeks, if this were the length of the grace period decided upon, they would not know if the baby they had contracted for would indeed remain with them or return to the surrogate. They, too, would ride an emotional roller coaster. They, too, would therefore require extensive psychological counseling before being permitted to enter into the contract. Yet it seems to me that their anguish, should the birth mother eventually decide to keep the child, would be intrinsically different from that of the woman who goes through a nine-month pregnancy and then must part with her baby. In the case of the couple contracting with a surrogate, bonding with the child has yet to occur. For the surrogate, it has already occurred, yet the contract must be honored in spite of this.

The counseling period recommended for both the surrogate mother—and her husband, if she is married—and the contracting couple prior to their entering into any agreement would also allow both parties to form a trusting relationship with those affording them counseling. Within the context of these separate relationships, hypothetical situations could be made concrete, anticipated emotions could be evoked immediately and the attempt be made to deal with them, and technical information could be placed into proper perspective.

Those providing the counseling could evaluate both the potential surrogate and the couple wishing to contract with her and make an assessment of the emotional stability and maturity of each. They could obtain informational feedback to assess the degree of understanding achieved by both parties, reach a judgment about the voluntariness of the contemplated arrangement, and explore the motivation of the surrogate. As has been pointed out, motivation may indeed be crucial to the whole enterprise: on a spectrum, the two ends of which might be termed "altruism" and "materialism," the closer the prospective surrogate comes to altruism, the more likely it is that the contract will be honored and the well-being of all parties assured.

Moral Concerns

These, then, are some of the moral concerns generated by surrogate motherhood: surrogacy for convenience, surrogacy commercialized, and the thorny problem of informed consent in this context. Against these qualms, we must balance compassion for childless couples who wish to achieve parenthood by this particular means. The legislative proposals which follow, tenuous as they are, reflect an attempt to do justice to both claims: that of the potential surrogate to be allowed to perform a largely altruistic service—a woman who has no difficulty conceiving undertaking to bear a child for her infertile sister—and that of the infertile couple to be afforded the opportunity to nurture a child of their own.

Legislation is necessary to place surrogate motherhood on a less ambiguous footing than that upon which it currently stands. Because of uneven policies in different states, it should be enacted at the federal level. It should constrain the capacity of Americans to circumvent its intentions by resort to surrogates in an international market. It should prohibit surrogacy for other than medical indications, difficult though these are to define with precision. It should provide for the mother's compensation for all legitimate medical expenses and for loss of earnings during her pregnancy, while eliminating the exorbitant brokerage fees paid to intermediaries. It should attempt to meet the complex moral and legal expectations of informed consent by requiring, for both parties to the contract, an extensive period of psychological counseling before entering into it. And it should allow a grace period during which the surrogate mother could change her mind about surrendering the baby she had borne and pay the requisite penalties for her breach of the initial agreement. With these provisions in place, surrogacy contracts should then be recognized as legally binding.

Bill and Barbara finally succeeded in having a baby of their own. Along the way to this happy outcome, during the darkest days of their apparent infertility, they explored at least one of the options the new reproductive technologies are now making available, that of in vitro *fertilization. How far along the spectrum of possibilities open to them they would have been willing to go would have depended very much on the level of their determination to have a child. Our task, as a society, is to balance with reason and compassion the values we cherish against their possible erosion because of the despair of childless couples and the readiness of some to exploit this for personal gain.*

Abortion

T*he entrances to family planning clinics are blocked by anti-abortionists,
so that neither the staff nor their clientele can enter the buildings.
Abortion clinics are bombed; there is extensive property damage, but
no one is hurt. Two Roman Catholic nuns finally resign from their order in
frustration over the Vatican's inflexible position on abortion and because of
harassment resulting from their principled dissent. The pros and cons of
federal and state funding for abortion are bitterly disputed. Despite sex
education programs in public schools, children continue to have children at
a catastrophically high rate. Presidential candidates are judged by the elec-
torate according to their stand on the abortion issue. Anti-abortion protesters
picket the White House. The exponential increase in global population, particularly in underdeveloped countries, threatens the ultimate survival of the
human race on planet earth. One in two pregnancies in the United States is
now aborted. In countries like Japan, abortion is the most popular means of
contraception. Christian leaders continue to denounce contraception as well
as abortion. These are but an arbitrarily selected few of a bewildering array
of facts surrounding the abortion controversy and continuing to inflame it.*

In the ongoing and emotionally volatile abortion debate, the protagonists are vehemently polarized and their positions clearly defined. There are, at one end of the spectrum, pro-life groups implacably opposed to abortion on moral grounds.[1] At the other, there are
pro-choice advocates unequivocally in favor of abortion on demand.[2]
Between these extremes, there are several mediating positions.[3]

My own views fall into the third category. I favor a liberal abortion law for the simple reason that restrictive laws are discriminatory (the wealthy can always fly their way around them) and dangerous (the poor will resort to back-street abortionists). At the same time, abortion is a morally complex issue, representing an often tragic choice of what appears to be the lesser of two evils rather than between absolutely right and wrong courses of action.

Pros and Cons

How is the problem of abortion best defined? To the extent that abortion is a medical procedure, it does present medical ethics with a subject to be addressed. But because abortion is often perceived by women confronting unintended, unexpected, or unwanted pregnancies to be the only realistic option available to them, this is ultimately a societal problem. How might a society afford such women positive, creative alternatives to abortion? So long as our society fails to address this fundamental issue, the topic continues to be diverted into the medical arena, where it may not properly, or permanently, belong.

Those whose views on abortion are diametrically opposed tend to be concerned with different sets of facts and are prone to discount the data not directly supportive of their respective positions. The pro-life wing concentrates almost exclusively on embryological and developmental facts to bolster its contention that the fetus is fully human from the moment of conception. In support of this claim, observations made by means of ultrasound sonography or fetoscopy are seen as crucial.[4] For the most part, those who adhere to the pro-choice position base their claims on facts pertaining to the mother: her age, level of education, marital status, number of dependents, sources of income, relationship to the child's father, need and ability to be independent, socioeconomic conditions, and overarching life goals.

Divergent values are espoused as well. The pro-life wing values the fetus as human from the moment of conception.[5] Proclaiming the fetus to be human from the moment of conception is indeed a value judgment; this is not an empirically demonstrable fact! And adherents to the pro-choice position value the woman's capacity to be self-determining and free from external constraints in matters of reproductive choice.[6]

The reasoning of each side is grounded in different assumptions. Typically, the pro-life argument is deontological. It is based on moral rules. Killing human beings is morally forbidden, *a priori*. Since fetuses are valued as human beings, abortion is not only wrong, it is the equivalent of murder.[7] (Curiously, the rule prohibiting killing is typically not extended to capital punishment or war!) Additionally, there is in the Judeo-Christian tradition a principle requiring the defense of the defenseless.[8] The fetus is the most vulnerable, the most defenseless party when abortion is being contemplated; therefore, the fetus must be defended even, and possibly especially, from the mother, whom the pro-choice advocates may characterize as herself acting in self-defense.

Commonly, the proponents of a pro-choice position reason consequentially. They are concerned with how individual women in particular circumstances would be affected in choosing among the various alternative courses of action open to them: carrying their babies to term and keeping them, carrying them to term and then giving them up for adoption, or terminating their pregnancies. In weighing these imagined but often predictable consequences, a decision is arrived at which will either minimize the harmful or maximize the beneficial results for the women directly concerned and sometimes for their husbands or lovers as well.[9]

Finally, both the pregnant women who contemplate having abortions and the medical caregivers who consider performing this procedure will act according to diverse perceived obligations. Some women will feel a primary obligation to their own well-being, regardless of the nascent life *in utero*. Others will feel an obligation to obey either their own conscience or the teachings of the religious communities to which they belong, discounting the adverse effects this might have on them personally. Some caregivers will feel an obligation to perform abortions as safely, competently, and nonjudgmentally as possible, regarding the women who come to them as their patients, whose needs are to be met expeditiously, effectively, confidentially, and compassionately. Others will feel obliged to take the side of the fetus, will refuse to be involved with abortions, and will usually refer patients to others whose conscience allows them to perform this procedure.

This analysis enables us to identify the many points of divergence and dispute between the protagonists in the abortion debate in terms of problem identification, the data they adduce and consider crucial, the values they uphold, the mode of reasoning they employ, and the obligations they deem primary. It thereby illustrates how descriptive ethics—the analysis of what is going on in a moral argument—proceeds. But what might normative ethics, concerned not with what is but with what ought to be happening, have to say about the moral quandary posed by abortion, and why?

Mediating Between Extremes: from Analysis to Prescription

My own normative position requires me to take account of all the relevant facts, not merely the data reckoned to be important by one side or the other.[10] Similarly, I am concerned both to value the fetus as at least potentially human from the moment of conception and to value the woman's need and capacity to be self-determining in matters of reproductive choice. No single value should arbitrarily be absolutized, to the exclusion of other values. I recognize the importance of the principles of preserving and protecting life and of defending the defenseless; at the same time, I cannot ignore a consideration of the consequences in looking at the particular options between which individual women must choose. And, as a caregiver, I feel a primary obligation to the woman who presents herself as a candidate for abortion, and only a secondary obligation to the potential human being *in utero*.

Accordingly, early in the pregnancy, I value the woman's need and capacity to be self-determining in terms of her reproductive choice more highly than I value the fetus as a potential human being. However, as the pregnancy proceeds and as the fetus becomes more recognizably human and more capable of surviving outside the womb, which is what is meant by the term "viability," I am compelled to reverse this ranking of values. In the absence of any diagnosed fetal malformation, the further advanced the pregnancy, the more I recognize the fetus's claim to life as being more important than the woman's reproductive choice.

As a caregiver, I would usually reckon myself to have a primary obligation to the woman rather than to the fetus. The professional obligation of the medical caregiver seems clear: the actual patient is primary; the fetus, who may also become a patient in the course of the interaction between the woman and her medical caregivers, is secondary. This view may be diagramed as shown in Figure 7-1.

Viability is that point, not when the fetus becomes human and is therefore entitled to the protection all other human beings enjoy, but when the fetus gains access to a support system other than the uterus, such as a neonatal intensive care unit. It is the availability of an

Figure 7-1: Diminishing and Increasing Rights of the Woman and the Fetus Respectively

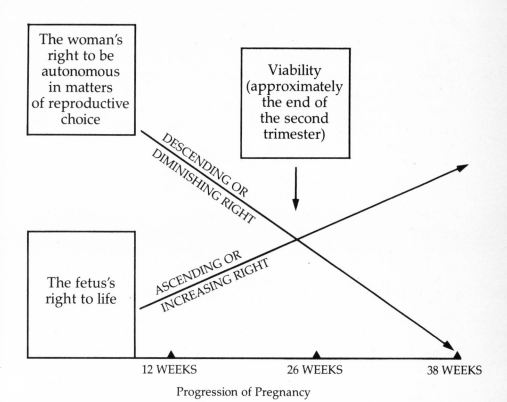

The woman's right to be autonomous in matters of reproductive choice

Viability (approximately the end of the second trimester)

DESCENDING OR DIMINISHING RIGHT

The fetus's right to life

ASCENDING OR INCREASING RIGHT

12 WEEKS   26 WEEKS   38 WEEKS

Progression of Pregnancy

alternative life support system that enables the state to exercise its interest in the protection of all human life, without unduly trespassing upon the woman's autonomy.

So long as a pregnancy cannot be terminated without killing the fetus, that is, prior to viability, I must accept with regret the death of the fetus as an often tragic necessity. But as soon as the pregnancy can be interrupted without the fetus necessarily being killed, as is the case in late-second- and early-third-trimester abortions, I feel obliged to make the attempt to preserve fetal life even as the pregnancy is terminated. Except in so-called therapeutic abortions, where fetal abnormalities have been diagnosed, making survival moot and the quality of the infants' survival, should they survive, incompatible with their own best interests, I do not believe that the woman's right to terminate a pregnancy necessarily includes a license to kill the fetus.

Parents do not own their children. Nor do they have an absolute right to dispose of them. Early on, the decision to terminate a pregnancy inevitably entails the killing of the fetus. But as viability approaches, these become, and should be regarded as, two separate issues. Now it becomes possible to insist on safeguarding the life of the abortus, even as the pregnancy is terminated. This point is crucial, for example, in deciding whether saline or prostaglandin should be used to accomplish the abortion; saline will kill the fetus, prostaglandin will not.[11]

As was seen in the previous chapter, techniques are now available for implanting an ovum that has been fertilized *in vitro* with sperm into the uterus either of the woman from whom the ovum was extracted—the genetic mother—or of a surrogate, who will become the biological mother. If these techniques of embryo implantation should be further refined, evolving to the point where it will become possible to perform this procedure, not merely at 4 to 5 days, but at 4 to 5 weeks, then terminating a pregnancy and killing a fetus could be regarded earlier on as two quite separate and distinguishable acts. The right to perform the one would no longer entail the necessity of the other. This technological development could lead to major changes in the law. Hypothetically, pregnancy termination would be legal; killing fetuses would not.

Should this possibility eventually be realizable, there might then be no losers in a situation where abortion is decided upon. The pregnant woman's need and capacity to be self-determining in reproductive choice could be honored. But, except in cases where it is established that the fetus is seriously abnormal or where no adoptive mother could be found, this would not give her license to kill the fetus. She might be required to surrender her abortus for implantation into the uterus of a surrogate mother, someone ready, willing, and able to carry the infant to term. Such a solution would meet the concerns of both the pro-life and pro-choice advocates. It would almost certainly reduce the number of abortions as well by compelling women contemplating abortion to weigh their proposed course of action even more seriously and carefully than is sometimes the case at present.

In the meantime, however, it is possible to satisfy one side in the abortion debate only at the expense of the other. Until fetuses are viable, life-support systems other than the uterus are not available to them. At the point at which infants can be kept alive in a neonatal intensive care unit, abortion is usually no longer legally permissible.

The normative approach just outlined seems, in the present circumstances, to offer the best solution to a dilemma fraught with complexity and resonant with elements of tragedy. It causes me to be a staunch advocate of a liberal abortion law, and at the same time to be committed to keeping alive the debate about abortion as a profound moral issue.

In Utero Diagnosis

Certain technologies are now providing us with new and highly accurate information about the fetus *in utero*, from very early in the pregnancy: ultrasound sonography, fetoscopy, and magnetic resonance imaging among them.[12] In a desired pregnancy, it is now not uncommon for a couple's collection of photographs of the new baby to begin with pictures taken *in utero*, by means of one or another of these new technologies. What effect might this have on the abortion controversy? It seems clear that it will strengthen the pro-life position, weaken that of advocates of pro-choice, and nudge increasing numbers of those subscribing to mediating positions toward the pro-life side of the spectrum.

The new imaging technologies will provide us with visual evidence of how akin to a human being a developing fetus is. This will cause the revulsion many feel to the taking of human life to be extended to include fetal life, if not at a few days of gestational age, then surely when the fetus is several weeks old. Pro-choice advocates will be driven more and more onto the defensive. They will be forced to face the question: How can a woman's emotional and socioeconomic well-being possibly be weighed on the same scale in any calculation of consequences which, for the developing fetus—someone who appears more and more to be a member of the human family—will mean certain death? Measured arguments will be required to give credence to a view that is likely to appear less and less tenable as factual evidence begins to accumulate in support of the contention that the developing fetus is an authentic member of the human community.

But it is upon those adhering to the mediating positions between the pro-choice and the pro-life extremes that the new imaging techniques will have the most profound effect, in two important ways. One will be a move in the direction of supporting third-trimester abortions in certain cases. A convincing moral case has been made recently for third-trimester abortions,[13] providing two conditions are fulfilled:

> a) the fetus is seen to be afflicted with a condition that either is incompatible with postnatal survival for more than a few weeks or is characterized by the total or virtual absence of cognitive function; and

> b) this determination is based on highly reliable diagnostic evidence.

In the opinion of those adopting this position, whereas "currently one entity, anencephaly [absence of the brain], clearly fulfills both conditions. . . . as antenatal sonography improves through technologic advances and increased clinical experience, other fetal disorders (for example, renal agenesis [failure of the kidneys to develop]) will probably join anencephaly in fulfilling both conditions."[14]

The moral argument is that in circumstances meeting the conditions prescribed, the termination of pregnancy may benefit pregnant women by reducing the period of time during which they would suffer the psychological pain of carrying a fetus with a hopeless prognosis. Termination may also benefit the parents by allowing them to initiate a subsequent pregnancy earlier than if the seriously abnormal pregnancy had been allowed to continue to term.

However, earlier in the gestational process, more precise imaging techniques applied with surer clinical experience may conceivably decrease the number of first-trimester abortions among those who take both embryological and fetal development and the woman's circumstances into account in reaching for a responsible decision. The pictorial evidence provided by the new imaging technologies that what is at stake in an abortion is the termination of what looks remarkably like a human life will work to the benefit of the fetus. It will be more difficult for a person whose conscience is sensitive on this score to proceed with a contemplated abortion, whether as a patient, a physician, or a nurse. Consequently, I am already on record as predicting that "the net effect of imaging technology will be to nudge the spectrum of ethical opinion on abortion considerably toward the right."[15]

Related Issues

Two further thorny issues must now be considered: one is engendered by the new genetics, the other by recent developments in the field of tissue and organ transplantation.

Identifying Inherited Diseases

Biochemists, as we have seen, are on the verge of being able to identify genetic markers for inherited diseases such as cystic fibrosis, cancer of the colon, and certain forms of breast cancer. Once this has been achieved, it will be possible to obtain fetal cells and to arrive at a diagnosis of major genetically related diseases early in the pregnancy, while it is both lawful and safe for a woman to have a therapeutic abortion. As we gain a more complete picture of which human genes are responsible for genetically related diseases, the number of inherited disorders that it will be possible to identify *in utero* will increase dramatically to something like 3,000. The quantity of fetuses who will then become candidates for abortion will expand concomitantly.

This will present new moral dilemmas. Is the fact that a female *in utero* will develop breast cancer when she is approximately 35 years of age sufficient reason for terminating both the pregnancy and her life? Is the fact that a male *in utero* will die of cystic fibrosis when he is approximately 30 years of age, unless a cure is discovered in the interim, and will have a life of uneven, but not devastatingly poor, quality until then, sufficient reason for performing a therapeutic abortion? As the number of diseases identifiable *in utero* by their genetic markers increases, which fetuses will not be candidates for therapeutic abortion, given the fact that departures from the genetic norm are commonplace and occur universally? None of us is without one or another genetic abnormality, however minor.

The argument might be made that aborting fetuses with identifiable genetically linked diseases at least allows the parents to attempt to have another normal child. But this begs the question: what is normal and who is to make this determination? If schizophrenia should turn out to be a genetically linked disease, as many now suspect it is, would this be a sufficient departure from the norm to warrant abortion? Would someone presently suffering from schizophrenia prefer not to have been born? And if schizophrenia warrants abortion, what about manic depression? Where does one draw the line? And ought the fact that both diseases can now be controlled pharmacologically militate against any decision to terminate such a pregnancy?

Furthermore, is it an entirely desirable goal to want to eliminate from the range of human experience the adversity and hardship associated with caring for a sickly child? I ask this question tentatively. I am well aware of the ways in which unalleviated suffering can devastate human beings, how the burden of an abnormal child can destroy families, and how much easier it is to bear other people's afflictions with equanimity than it is to respond to one's own creatively and with courage. Nevertheless, I cannot help wondering whether we human beings could ever really know joy if it were not for pain; whether we could ever truly understand the meaning of love if it were not for the ways in which others stand with us when we are afflicted by cruel and unusual circumstances; whether we could ever completely appreciate the light were there not also seasons of darkness. Therefore, I am not convinced that the elimination, as distinct from the alleviation, of suffering is a desirable goal for the human species— let alone one capable of attainment.

Between those at one end of a spectrum who are as close to being genetically normal as it is possible to be and those at the other who are grossly abnormal, there is a wide grey zone. One way of helping couples with an affected fetus whose condition puts it into this area of ambiguity to make a responsible decision about whether or not to abort may be suggested. It is that of encouraging them to consult with parents of children with the same condition, as well as with those presently burdened with the same disease, before proceeding with a contemplated abortion. Such consultation need not constrain their eventual choice; it could, however, serve to inform it.

Fetal Transplants

Another vexing moral problem associated with abortion is the use of aborted fetal cells or organs or tissue for purposes of transplantation. Medical scientists have recently sought to reverse the progressive neurological deterioration caused by Parkinson's disease, for example, by transplanting fetal brain cells into the brains of patients with this disease. The results are highly promising. Apparently, fetal brain cells continue to grow, thus rejuvenating the brain of the host. They are not susceptible to rejection in the same way that the cells of an adult or even a child would be. There is concern, however, about the moral propriety of using fetuses as means to other ends, however laudable these ends may be in and of themselves.

It is important to distinguish between the use of spontaneously or selectively aborted fetuses, on the one hand, and, on the other, of fetuses conceived and aborted with the sole intention that their cells or organs will then be sold. The former, if handled with sensitivity and respect, can provide bereaved parents with some sense of meaning in what may otherwise be a meaningless event—the consolation of knowing that the baby they wanted but could not have is helping someone else to live normally or better. The latter blatantly uses fetuses instrumentally and raises the specter of "fetal farms"—fetuses grown and then aborted for commercial reasons. This ought never to be condoned. It diminishes the humanity of all of us.

One way of approaching the issue of fetal transplantation would be to agree, at the outset, that it falls into the category of investigational or experimental medicine, rather than that of established therapeutics. Once this distinction is made, then the norms governing research can be invoked. These would include preliminary work *in vitro* (in the laboratory), proceeding to *in vivo* studies of animals whose physiology, in relevant respects, resembles that of the human species. Only when the results of these preliminary investigations were favorable enough to warrant the next major step could the transplantation of fetal material into human recipients be contemplated. (In the United States this is presently prohibited; fetal tissue transplants are being done beyond, but not within, our borders.)

Centers could be identified where, on the basis of an established record of successful laboratory and animal work, the knowledge gained could be fruitfully employed in experimental transplantations. It would be necessary to submit proposals for research involving fetal organs or tissue to the review boards of selected institutions. The design of the experiments and what they were intended to accomplish would need to be described in detail.

Federal approval for proceeding would also be required. Then, and only then, could the collaboration of couples about to abort a pregnancy with potential recipients or their parents be solicited. This collaboration would be subject to the standards of fully informed and substantially voluntary consent and refusal. Only when statistically significant data had been accumulated demonstrating the safety and efficacy of the experimental procedures could a move from the investigational to the clinical setting be envisioned.

At this juncture, federal regulation would be necessary to guard against a widespread loss of respect for fetal life. Guidelines would need to be drawn up specifying the circumstances in which normal aborted fetuses or tissue taken from them could be used for transplantation purposes, and how this would be regulated. The moral and legal requirements of informed consent would have to be satisfied by both donors and recipients or their surrogates. And the decent and respectful disposition of the fetal remains would have to be assured. Only with these provisos is it remotely possible to consider using fetuses or fetal tissue to serve therapeutic ends—however worthy in themselves these ends might be. The Kantian categorical imperative still haunts us: always treat human beings as ends, and never merely as a means.

Teenage Parenthood

A final quandary relative to abortion may be mentioned: children having children. When a fourteen- or fifteen-year-old girl, still living at home and almost totally dependent on her parents' emotional and financial support, finds herself with an unplanned or unwanted pregnancy, what role, if any, ought her parents to have in her decision whether or not to have an abortion? There are times when such a fourteen- or fifteen-year-old will not want to abort her baby, while her parents, perhaps with a more realistic view of her chances of attaining a good life in this society without having completed her high school education, are insisting that she terminate the pregnancy. And, conversely, there are times when the teenager will want an abortion because she sees having a baby as interfering too radically with her life plans, while her parents wish her to continue with the pregnancy, promising to afford her all necessary support before and after the child is born to enable her to resume her life as uninterruptedly as possible. To what extent ought parental wishes to intrude on the autonomous choice of a fourteen- or fifteen-year-old, especially where the parents are willing and able to shoulder responsibility, financial and otherwise, for the choice they are insisting on?

The autonomy of adolescents is a complex issue. We have no agreed-upon societal standard of transition from minor to adult. If she is given permission to marry, a fourteen- or fifteen-year-old is regarded as an emancipated minor. At sixteen, adolescents in some states can obtain a driver's license—something akin to the initiation rites prevalent in tribal cultures. At eighteen, young men and women can fight, and die, for their country; yet, in most states, they may not purchase beer until they turn twenty-one.

A seventeen-year-old recently sailed singlehandedly around the world; many twenty-seven-year-olds (and forty-seven-year-olds!) are not nearly as mature. Thirteen-year-olds, stricken with a terminal disease, often become wise and mature beyond their years and are responsibly involved in decisions about whether or not to receive further therapy. What, then, is the physician to do when confronted with a young teenager, still dependent on her parents, whose wishes either to carry a pregnancy to term or to terminate it are being opposed by them?

It is the pregnant fourteen- or fifteen-year-old, not her parent, who is the patient in this particular relationship between patient and physician. It is with her that the physician has a primary connection; any relationship the physician may have with the pregnant patient's parents is secondary. It is important that this be recognized and remembered, however dependent on her parents the fourteen- or fifteen-year-old may be. In each particular situation, the physician must attempt to discern how capable the pregnant teenager is of making an informed and responsible choice.

If, in the physician's judgment, the teenager is mature enough to understand what she is about, it is then necessary to proceed to make every effort to discern what the patient, rather than her parents, wants, and to become her advocate in dealing with her parents. The mere fact that the physician becomes the pregnant adolescent's advocate can often provide a catalyst for family discussions less emotionally charged than they might otherwise be. The physician's advocacy may not be successful in terms of having the teenager's wishes prevail over those of her parents. But it may be regarded as successful either if she decides to follow her own heart rather than the advice of her parents, having often listened to their point of view; or if she decides to follow the advice of her parents rather than her own heart, after they have listened to her expressions of opinion.

In cases where the physician becomes convinced that the teenager is too immature to be capable of making informed and responsible decisions, his obligation will be different. Now it will consist of attempting to educate the pregnant girl about the consequences of the various options between which she has to choose. It may further consist of reinforcing parental expressions of opinion if these seem genuinely to reflect the best interests of the teenager rather than their own convenience.

Parental support, or the lack of it, is a crucial variable in any teenage girl's decision whether to abort a pregnancy or to carry it to term. Nevertheless, parental support is not ultimately the crucial factor. What is decisive is that it is principally her life that will be affected one way or the other by her choosing whether or not to have an abortion. The physician's obligation is to help keep her in a central decision-making role, with the likelihood of parental support or lack of it providing some of the data necessary for an informed choice. The physician's role as advocate is also that of helping to prevent her from being emotionally blackmailed by her parents. Only in cases where the teenager is markedly immature, and where the judgment of the parents seems to be sound, does it behoove the physician to reinforce their beneficent and well-intentioned paternalism.

Here, as in so many other areas of medicine, prevention is better than cure. Frank and open discussion about sexuality in the home, coupled with parental willingness to provide contraceptive advice and choice to their sexually active teenage children, is infinitely preferable to after-the-fact, traumatic decisions about abortion. Perhaps the single most important prerequisite for this is for those of us who are parents to stop denying that our children are sexual, and often sexually active, human beings.

8

Perinatology

Even as I write, I am called to the emergency room to be with Debbie, a young mother whose baby is dying. I leave my computer and go at once to the hospital. Debbie is 21 years old, black, unmarried, and already has a five-year-old son. She was in the seventh month of her pregnancy. For the past eight months, she has been a street person. She and her son have slept in abandoned cars and buildings, and in vacant lots. The local ecumenical hunger program has supplied them with food. Her parents are both dead. Yesterday, her uncle died—of diabetes and cancer. This threw her into a paroxysm of grief, which brought on labor. This morning, she delivered prematurely. Paramedics called to the scene resuscitated the infant girl. Too tiny and too weak to survive until admission to the intensive care nursery, she died in the emergency room. She, too, will become an infant mortality statistic. I am angry because I believe that had her mother received adequate food, housing, and prenatal care, the baby might have lived.

Perinatology? The word has an esoteric ring to it. It is not yet to be found in Webster's. Literally, it means "surrounding (peri) the newborn (the neonate)." It refers to the work of neonatologists—pediatricians practicing their healing art in the highly technological and sophisticated environment of modern newborn intensive care units—and the obstetricians who collaborate with them in identifying high-risk pregnancies and treating the women concerned and the babies they carry before rather than after delivery.

As a subspecialty of pediatrics, neonatology is a mere fifteen or twenty years old. It has been only within the last decade that neonatologists and obstetricians have begun to work together closely in diagnosing, *in utero*, problems likely to affect babies after birth, and in bringing the mothers to neonatal intensive care centers to deliver, thus making possible more effective treatment.

There are three categories of infants requiring intensive care. First, there are those who are born prematurely and/or are small for gestational age. Obstetricians can be helpful in identifying pregnant women at risk for giving birth to such babies; many of these women are young, impoverished, addicted to alcohol or street drugs, malnourished, in poor physical health, or have been treated with fertility drugs. Debbie's story is typical of those that could be told about mothers and their babies in this category.

Second, there are children born with congenital abnormalities. Among these, for example, are:

> *Down's syndrome*—characterized by mental deficiency, physical abnormalities, and a higher-than-normal susceptibility to infection
> *spina bifida cystica* (also known as myelomeningocele or meningomyelocele)—a major neural tube defect consisting of a cystic lesion on the back resulting in paralysis below the lesion
> *hydrocephalus*—a progressive enlargement of the head from increased amounts of cerebrospinal fluid in the ventricles of the brain which, if untreated, can lead to permanent brain damage
> *hydroencephaly*—the complete or almost complete absence of the cerebral hemispheres
> *anencephaly*—a condition of arrested development of the brain in which at least one of the cerebral hemispheres is absent, and sometimes the entire brain
> *hypoplastic left heart syndrome (or other heart diseases)*—incomplete development of the vessels on the left side of the heart, preventing the circulation of oxygenated blood
> *trisomy 18*—characterized by profound mental deficiency, difficulty in breathing, low birthweight, and severe gastrointestinal and renal deformities
> *trisomy 13*—this condition results in the incomplete development of the forebrain, severe mental deficiency, major eye abnormalities, and congenital heart disease

diaphragmatic hernia—a protrusion of the abdominal organs into the thoracic cavity through an opening in the diaphragm, often found in infants with Down's syndrome
exstrophy of the cloaca—in neonates having no cloacal membrane, the common passage for fecal, urinary, and reproductive discharge is turned inside out
De Lange syndrome—severe mental deficiency, congenital heart disease, excessive facial and body hair, and limb reduction
Apert's syndrome—a condition involving the premature fusion of the cranial sutures, mental retardation, and webbing of the hands and feet
Lesch-Nyhan syndrome—a recessive disease linked to the X chromosome involving a process of neurological and physiological deterioration from approximately the sixth month of life; the most striking feature of the syndrome is compulsive self-mutilation
Tay-Sachs disease—another recessive condition occurring with higher than normal frequency among Ashkenazic Jews, with symptoms appearing about six months after birth and signaling an inexorable decline of mental and physical ability until death occurs at about three or four.

Obstetrician-gynecologists are often able to diagnose such problems *in utero* and, in cases where the mothers do not elect to have therapeutic abortions, make arrangements ahead of time for them to deliver their babies at neonatal intensive care centers.

The third category comprises full-term, normal infants who sustained some untoward and traumatic event in the birth process: the umbilical cord wrapped around the baby's neck, for example, cutting off the oxygen supply to the brain. Such infants usually require resuscitation and then intubation—having a tube which is connected to a breathing machine inserted into the windpipe—so that they can be ventilated mechanically. Some of them are later discovered to have sustained brain damage.

Perinatology now commands approximately $2.6 billion of the total spent annually on American health care. In the relatively short time that it has been accepted and integrated into modern medicine, impressive advances have occurred. With respect to low-birthweight premature infants, for example, the infants' potential for survival keeps being pushed back to lower and lower limits: from 2,000 grams to 1,500 grams, from 1,500 grams to 1,000 grams, from 1,000 grams to 750 grams, and from 750 grams to 500 grams and less (traditionally, weights of infants in neonatal intensive care units are given in grams rather than pounds; a pound is equal to a little less than 500 grams). These bare facts conceal remarkable technological accomplishments. Both the science and the art of perinatology are becoming ever surer. This stems as much from advances in nursing and bioengineering as from gains in medicine itself.

Nevertheless, there is a dark side to all of this. The infant mortality rate in this country grows worse rather than better. And many of the babies rescued in our neonatal intensive care units survive with delays, deficits, or disabilities. The morbidity range is from mild, to moderate, to profound impairment. Such morbidity is often attributable to the very technology which cheated death. That is to say, it is iatrogenic in nature—from the Greek words *iatros*, physician, and *genesis*, originating. The harm is inflicted by the very treatments that are intended to preserve life.

A recent article in the *New England Journal of Medicine* contains a table which illustrates this point with respect to very low-birthweight premature infants. It includes data from six different sources for approximately the same period. An abbreviated version of the table follows.

Table 8-1: Survival and Neurodevelopmental Outcome of Extremely Small Infants*

Year of Birth	Birth Weight (in grams—500 g = approx. 1 lb.)	Survived to Discharge (%)	Neurodevelopmental Handicap (%)
1977–1980	500–800	29	34
1977–1980	500–800	20	25
1977–1981	500–800	44	35
1977–1980	500–750	42	27
1975–1980	500–750	40	32
1982–1984	500–750	26	33

*Source: Extracted from material originally appearing in Maureen Hack, M.B., Ch.B., and Avroy A. Fanaroff, M.B., F.R.C.P. (E.), D.C.H., "Special Report: Changes in the Delivery Room Care of the Extremely Small Infant (750 g): Effects on Morbidity and Outcome," *New England Journal of Medicine*, vol. 314, no. 10, March 6, 1986, pp. 660–664.

Recent data from our own neonatal intensive care nursery at Stanford corroborate these disquieting statistics: in the 500 to 750-gram birthweight category, approximately 25 percent of the infants survive; of these, only about 70 percent are normal. Such are some of the questionable triumphs of contemporary technology.

Besides being extremely expensive, the fact that perinatology is a not unmixed blessing gives rise to several of the ethical conundrums which confront neonatologists and obstetricians as well as those who are concerned with the moral implications of contemporary medicine. These may be conceptualized best by means of a diagram (see Figure 8-1).

The infant is at the center of the triangle, the focus of much care and attention on the part of the participants in the drama of the newborn intensive care nursery. At the top corner of the triangle is the perinatal team. It is comprised of neonatologists, obstetricians, and, depending on the level of intensive care being offered, support services such as cardiology, cardiac surgery, neurology, neurosurgery, nephrology, gastroenterology, and hematology; fellows, residents, in-

Figure 8-1: Principals in Neonatal Intensive Care and the Relationships Between Them

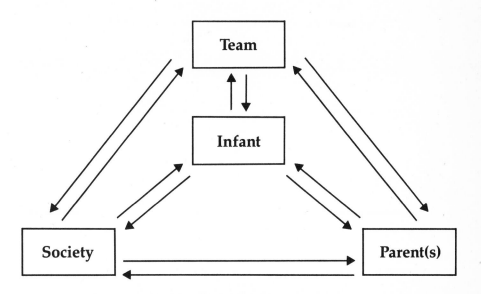

terns, and medical students; neonatal intensive care nurses; social workers, chaplains, and, in some centers, a resident ethics consultant.

There can be few areas in medicine where a team approach is more in evidence than in perinatology. The level of consultation and collaboration between physicians of various specialties and between physicians and ancillary health care providers is remarkably high. The team is primarily responsible, in consultation with the parents, for deciding what medical interventions are to be applied, withheld, or withdrawn for the benefit of the infant; for interpreting the results of such actions; and for constantly reappraising the treatment plan.

The parent or parents are at the second corner of the triangle. Often a young mother is the only parent, the father of the child having left her before or after the baby was born. Even when the father and mother are still together, one parent frequently stays with the baby in the hospital while the other remains at home, taking care of the other children. Regional neonatal intensive care nurseries may be at the center of a referral area up to one hundred fifty miles in radius. For most parents, having a baby in an intensive care nursery is a new and frightening experience; they are unprepared to move with any confidence in this strange, sophisticated world of biomedical technology. Also, they are often in shock. And not infrequently the ethnic, cultural, and language group to which they belong is very different from that of the predominantly Anglo team. Parents require, and generally receive, enormous emotional and spiritual support as they care for their infants in the neonatal nursery.

Society is represented at the third corner of the triangle. Third-party providers—Medicare, MediCal, private insurers, or agencies such as Crippled Children's Services—for the most part meet the extraordinarily high costs of neonatal intensive care. Seldom are these costs borne directly by the parents themselves. The law must be included at this end of the triangle as well: judges who will act speedily to provide injunctions requiring or restraining treatment, courts deciding in particular cases, legislators, and regulators. When neonatal intensive care began to flourish in the late 1960s, this corner of the triangle was at some considerable distance removed from the other two. But the costs and consequences of neonatal intensive care can no longer be ignored by society; therefore, it has moved steadily toward the equilateral position.

Ethical issues are generated as the team interacts with the infant and deals with the parent or parents, and as society impinges on the team.

The Team and the Infant:
Treatment or Nontreatment

Where there is a perinatal team of obstetricians collaborating with neonatologists rather than working independently of them, decisions about treatment and selective nontreatment can begin *in utero*. With data obtained from amniocentesis, chorionic villae sampling (whereby fetal cells, rather than merely fetal urine, can be scrutinized), and/or the new imaging technologies, obstetricians are now able to diagnose medical problems affecting fetuses while they are still in the womb.

Some of these, such as the failure of the ureters to drain urine from the kidneys to the bladder, may be amenable to surgical correction. Research done with primates, and on a limited basis with human fetuses, suggests that it is possible to remove developing infants from the uterus, perform the corrective surgery safely, return them to the womb, and allow the pregnancies to proceed normally to term. The question to be weighed, not only by perinatologists but by society at large, is whether or not this is desirable from a medical, moral, and economic standpoint.

Fetal surgery provides an example of yet another intrusion into natural processes. Many of the candidates for fetal surgery would otherwise be stillborn. In terms of Darwinian selection, the principle of the survival of the fittest would take its relentless toll. In rescuing such infants, otherwise doomed to die, what are we doing to the gene pool? In expending shrinking resources on such heroic feats, are we diverting necessary funding away from preventive measures such as prenatal care, which many believe to be the single most necessary step to be taken if our national infant mortality statistics are to be improved? And how do we come to grips with the moral irony of such dramatic interventions for some fetuses, while we continue fairly casually to abort so many others of equal gestational age and with better prospects for survival? These are but some of the ethical questions raised by fetal surgery.

Once an infant has been born and after resuscitation has been brought into an intensive care nursery, the team begins to confront a series of questions, all of which have far-reaching ethical ramifications: What is the goal of intensive care? Merely survival to the point where the baby will be able to go home? Or does the quality of the infant's survival also matter?

This last question has become exceedingly vexing in the wake of the so-called Baby Doe Regulations, the background of which may not be generally well known. In 1982, an infant, Baby Doe, died in Bloomington, Indiana, after his parents refused corrective surgery for birth defects accompanying Down's syndrome. Within weeks, on President Reagan's instructions, the Secretary of Health and Human Services (HHS) notified health care providers that Section 504 of the Rehabilitation Act of 1973, which prohibits discrimination on the basis of handicap, should be applied to the treatment of infants with disabilities. Because there had been insufficient opportunity for public review and comment, the courts rejected this first Baby Doe Rule.

In 1984, after inviting and receiving views from concerned citizens over the period of time prescribed by law, HHS published its final version of the Baby Doe Rule. This was followed by the related Child Abuse Amendments of 1984 and the Child Abuse Rule of 1985, both of which attempted more closely to define the terms of the Baby Doe Regulations and the exceptions to their requirements. The federal Baby Doe Regulations attempted a heavy-handed resolution of subtle moral quandaries, requiring all infants, except those for whom this would obviously have been futile, to be treated aggressively. Not to do so would have rendered the attending physicians culpable of both child neglect and discrimination against the handicapped. All "quality of life" considerations were expressly disallowed as part of the decision-making process.

Unfortunately, while this simplistic approach solved dilemmas within the setting of the newborn nursery, it created further problems for the parents of survivors once the babies were discharged from the hospital and taken home. Many infants whom neonatologists were now obliged to treat aggressively survived with moderate to profound disabilities. At the very time such doubtful accomplishments were being mandated, the federal government was cutting back on resources available for the care of the handicapped. Subsequently, the Supreme Court of the United States declared the Baby Doe Rule invalid. However, the Child Abuse Amendments of 1984 and the Child Abuse Rule of 1985 remain law, although their force and the interpretation they are given may be affected by the invalidation of the Baby Doe Rule.

This failed attempt by the federal government had been designed specifically to exclude "quality of life" considerations from the decision-making process. The Child Abuse Amendments and the Child Abuse Rule obviously still have a bearing on decisions whether or not to escalate neonatal technology on the one hand, or to withhold or withdraw it on the other. And when there is uncertainty both about the likelihood of survival and, should babies survive, the degree to which they will have been either helped or harmed, the difficulties confronting the team are exacerbated. We shall consider these problems in turn.

Which Damaged Newborns Should be Saved?

The report of the President's commission, *Deciding to Forego Life-Sustaining Treatment*,[1] identified three broad categories of seriously ill newborns. At one end of the spectrum are those for whom intensive therapy clearly would be beneficial. Most neonatologists would agree that the Down's syndrome infant, as an example, falls into this group. At the opposite end of the spectrum are those for whom intensive care obviously would be futile, the children born without brains or kidneys, for example. And in between would be those for whom aggressive interventions would have ambiguous or uncertain results. In this group we might have the very-low-birth-weight infant, the child born with *spina bifida*, or the baby who had sustained brain damage due to intracranial bleeding or *anoxia* (the cutting off of the brain's oxygen supply).

The principle of *beneficence* dictates that in the first category, everything possible should be done for the infant. Equally, the principle of *nonmaleficence* dictates that where aggressive interventions would in any case be futile (the second category), the infant should not be harmed by being subjected to them and should be allowed to die naturally and peacefully. It is in the third group, where the harms and benefits of treatment are uncertain and ambiguous, that decision making becomes tragically difficult. Here, the delicacy and precision of the scalpel is required of those who must make life-or-death decisions; the Baby Doe Regulations swept all moral and medical scruples aside with the force of a bulldozer.

Although these regulations were subsequently struck down by the Supreme Court, many neonatologists are understandably nervous about invoking "quality of life" as a decision-making criterion. Quality-of-life decisions are most acceptable when what this phrase means is defined by conscious, adult patients themselves, as they evaluate their present or projected circumstances. When patients are unable either to define the phrase for us, or to invoke it with reference to their present or anticipated level of functioning, it becomes problematic in the extreme. Such is the case with unconscious or incompetent adults and with newborns.

For this reason, many are turning away from quality of life as an explicit decision-making criterion. The term has become so loaded emotionally that other criteria for decision-making in the zone of ambiguity or uncertainty are being explored—a necessary step if we do not subscribe to the notion that physical life, irrespective of its texture, its capacities for autonomy and for relating and responding to other human beings, has an absolute value and should be upheld at any cost.

The principle of *nonmaleficence*, summed up in the dictum *primum non nocere*—first of all, or above all else, do no harm—affords a guideline that can be helpfully applied to many cases in the ambiguous category. All interventions produce a certain amount of harm to the infant. One has only to watch a newborn child protesting the insertion of an intravenous line to realize this! Usually, the harm is minimal and is justified by the large, hoped-for ensuing benefits. But when the harm-benefit ratio shifts clearly in the direction of fewer benefits and greater harm, then surely the time has come when withdrawing or withholding heroic interventions must be considered.

Inevitably, those who care for seriously ill newborns—the team and the parents—have to use subjective indicators for assessing harm. There are few, if any, objective means of quantifying an infant's pain. But there is a point in the treatment of many infants when both the team and the family spontaneously recognize that not only are the treatments ineffective, but that the infants are being tortured. At this point, the principle of nonmaleficence requires that aggressive interventions be withheld or withdrawn, and that the babies be allowed a natural death—preferably at home and in their parents' arms.

The very-low-birthweight infant (in the 500 to 750-gram or one-and-a-quarter to one-and-a-half-pound range) presents a particularly complicated set of problems. As we have already seen, only 25 percent of such infants survive, and of these, about 30 percent are impaired. In the face of such statistics, how ought the team to treat the particular 500-gram infant who is brought into the neonatal intensive care unit?

Criteria for Treating Damaged Newborns

Nancy Rhoden, associate professor of law at Ohio State University, has an interesting cross-cultural perspective on this issue.[2] Her research in the United States, Sweden, and Britain led her to identify three alternative approaches to prognostic uncertainty. The *wait until certainty* approach appears to be predominant in our own country. Choosing to err on the side of life rather than death, and placing a high value on actual individual lives—and less value on anonymous statistical lives—we tend always to treat individual infants aggressively until it becomes absolutely certain that they either will not survive or are being gravely harmed. It is "a policy that focuses on the worst potential outcome and avoids it at all costs." This strategy maximizes "the number of infants who die slowly over weeks or months, as well as the number who live, but in a hopelessly impaired condition." Rhoden believes that the doctors who follow it "will increasingly be governed by technology instead of employing it as a tool," and that the parents' role is reduced to that of "onlookers." Needless to say, it is a strategy which consumes enormous resources.

At the opposite end of the scale is what Rhoden calls *the statistical prognostic strategy* typical of Sweden. This approach "does not regard the death of an individual infant who could have been saved as the worst type of error"; instead, it "seeks to minimize the number of infants who die slow deaths or who live with profound handicaps, and is willing to sacrifice some potentially 'good' survivors to achieve this goal."

Because the Swedes have addressed the major socioeconomic causes of prematurity, the number of very-low-birthweight premature infants in Sweden is approximately five times less, per capita, than it is in the United States. There are no slums in Sweden, and pregnant women are well fed, adequately housed, and afforded the best possible prenatal care. Second, Swedish society is relatively small and predominantly homogeneous, whereas ours is manifestly larger and heterogeneous. A societal consensus about values and priorities is therefore more readily attainable there than here. And, third, the Swedish form of socialism tends to place less emphasis on the individual and his rights and more on the common good than is the case in our own individualistic and competitive society. These comments are offered as caveats. They explain why the Swedish approach would never be adopted as normative in the United States.

But what we might move toward adopting is the third approach identified by Rhoden, what she calls *the individualized prognostic strategy* to be discerned in Britain. It is a time-limited way of proceeding, used "only in situations where continuing treatment indefinitely will mean, in practice, that even the most profoundly impaired infants will survive." It avoids the extremes of "either treating all infants until the outcome is certain or withholding treatment because the infant is in a class where the prognosis is grim." Neither outcome is to be avoided at all costs: either sacrificing potentially salvageable infants, which is possible in Sweden, or saving those who will be severely impaired, as happens in the United States.

British doctors err in both directions, though "they seek, through clinical observations, to minimize each type of mistake." Their approach relies heavily on constant re-evaluation and re-assessment of treatment decisions; it also conserves scarce resources, though this is not the motive for adopting it. It also involves the parents extensively in the decision-making process. Where, at the outset, both the benefits and harms of neonatal intensive care are uncertain, it suggests a medically, morally, and economically responsible treatment plan.

Pushing the Limits

We move on to a related moral issue: ECMO, or extra-corporeal membrane oxygenation.[3] Infants born with a congenital diaphragmatic hernia have, at best, a one-in-five chance of survival. Such infants are commonly classified as "responders" and "nonresponders," depending on whether or not their pulmonary artery pressures respond to the drugs used to bring them down, or to contrived changes in blood gas concentrations. The mortality rate for those who do not respond is greater than 80 percent. It is for such poor-prognosis infants that ECMO offers some hope as a treatment of last resort. But there is a catch to all this. The preferred form of the technology carries with it a high risk of inducing brain damage in the infants it is instrumental in saving.

Many neonatal intensive care centers have rushed headlong into deploying this new technology with predictably mixed results. Initially, the team at Stanford, recognizing that this is an experimental approach, proceeded more cautiously. Research protocols were drawn up so that the neonatal staff could learn to use ECMO with animals, observing the results, both good and bad. Only later was the next step to have been taken: employing ECMO in carefully designed and controlled experiments with human subjects. Some are of the opinion that we are not yet ready for this advance; yet the decision has been made to forge ahead. One hopes that the proposed intervention will not yet be presented to the parents as a "therapeutic" option and that it will be offered for what it is, an investigational procedure. As such, it will require their enlistment as collaborators in an experiment, rather than their concurrence in applying to their infants an established beneficial therapeutic modality.

Some Stanford neonatologists believe that a similar approach ought to characterize the treatment of the very-low-birthweight premature infant. Instead of presenting intensive care of such tiny infants (<750 grams) as therapeutic, which, on the basis of the statistics already quoted, is obviously an exaggeration, it ought to be reclassified as investigational. The justification for experimenting at the frontiers of viability is that, inevitably, lessons are learned that can save the lives of larger and more mature infants. Parents could choose whether or not to enlist their very tiny premature infants in such investigational protocols after being made aware of the potential risks and benefits both of neonatal intensive care itself and of the alternatives, which are not many, available to them. But they would not be giving consent to established therapeutic interventions. Only as the data warrant subsequent reclassification from investigational to therapeutic could this begin to happen.

Such a strategy would achieve several important goals. It would truthfully represent the state of the art, which, at the frontiers, is investigational rather than therapeutic. It would involve the parents in what is actually happening to their infants: they are being volunteered as participants in research; they are not being afforded conventional care. And it would conserve society's shrinking resources. The amount spent on research would not be nearly as much as that currently being expended on therapy. And when a shift was made to greater therapeutic expenditures, it could be on the basis of solid data and represent a societal decision. Such an approach would provide a fourth alternative to the three identified by Nancy Rhoden.

Using Infants As Organ Donors

Before leaving the infant corner of the triangle, a further ethical issue might be mentioned briefly: that of using anencephalic (brain-absent) children as organ donors. There is before the

California Legislature at present Assembly Bill No. 2770. The section of the bill relevant to our concerns reads as follows:

> Notwithstanding any other provision of law, no person shall provide any life-sustaining procedure, as defined in Section 7187, to an infant born with anencephaly to temporarily prolong the infant's life so that the body or any part of the infant may be used for the purpose of transplantation.

The bill appears to have been designed expressly to thwart the Loma Linda Medical Center's recently suspended neonatal heart transplantation program, as well as others that might be inaugurated in its wake. At Loma Linda, there was a departure from standard medical practice in the way anencephalic babies were treated. Normally such babies are not afforded intensive care—ventilatory support or other mechanical and pharmacological means to prolong the inevitable process of dying. At Loma Linda, where such babies were seen as potential organ donors, their dying was vigorously prolonged by artificial means so as to preserve in the best possible condition the organs that were to be harvested from them.

What this amounted to is that these babies were treated not as ends in themselves, but as means to other ends. This is not merely unethical; it sets a bad precedent for the practice of medicine. The counterargument, that brain-dead adults also have their dying prolonged by artificial means so that they can provide fresh organs for transplantation, does not bear close scrutiny. Usually, in the adult, artificial life-sustaining means are applied initially in the hope of extending life and before brain death has been declared. Once brain death has been determined, and the family have agreed that organs may be donated, the artificial life-support systems are kept in place until the transplant surgery begins.

This is entirely different from maintaining brain-absent infants on life-support systems not for their own sake but for the sake of others who could benefit from the organs they provide. For this reason, I wholeheartedly support Assembly Bill No. 2770. To keep alive the anencephalic infant for potential use as an organ donor not only treats the brain-absent individual as a means to an end, it diminishes the humanity of those who resort to such means, however laudable their objectives may be. There is a moral difference between using the living and the dead as organ donors; it ought not to be blurred.

Interaction Between the Parents and the Team

I n most modern neonatal intensive care nurseries, the parent or parents are encouraged to be actively involved in bonding with the infant. Gone are the days when they were allowed into the nursery only at visiting hours. They are made to feel welcome around the clock, and are invited to be directly involved in the feeding, medicating, and nurturing of their babies.

But their role does not end there. More and more, the team attempts to enroll the parents as participants in the process of making decisions about what form care for their infants should take. At times, parents may feel that more should be done for their babies than the team may believe to be warranted on the basis of the available data. On other occasions, the converse may apply: parents want less to be done for their infants than the team deems necessary. And, when the parents live at some considerable distance away from where their baby is being treated and have other siblings to provide for, their consent for procedures to be performed often has to be obtained indirectly, over the telephone, rather than in person and face to face. This, coupled with the parents' grief and their possibly different ethnic background from that of the caregivers, gives rise to major difficulties with respect to informed consent. We shall consider these three issues in turn.

Parents Wanting Too Much Treatment

Recently, a very-low-birthweight, extremely premature infant was transported to our intensive care nursery from a city more than a hundred miles away, where the parents lived. As so often happens when an infant's lungs are too immature to exchange blood gases, the requisite ventilatory support further damaged the lungs, rendering the baby chronically ventilator-dependent. After four or five months in the nursery, it was apparent to all members of the treating team that this infant was not going to get well, and that he was being tortured rather than treated, harmed more than he was being helped. Unanimously, all members of the team became convinced that the time had come to stop caring aggressively for this baby, and to start caring palliatively for him while allowing him to have a natural death.

The parents, however, had extremely dogmatic and idiosyncratic religious views. So far as we could determine, they did not belong to any established religious community, but they claimed to have had a direct promise from God that their child would be healed. They came to the medical center only infrequently, due to their family responsibilities at home, and when they did come, they invariably insisted that their baby was improving, despite the evidence before their eyes and the protests of the staff that he was in agony as a result of the treatments he was receiving. Whenever any member of the team ventured to suggest that possibly the time had come to think about withdrawing aggressive therapy so that their baby could die naturally and peacefully, they expressed outrage. This would violate their agreement with God, based on the promise they believed themselves to have been given. And in the meantime the cost of their infant's care, which was being borne by MediCal, was well over $500,000.

The team felt frustrated in the extreme. As one of the attending neonatologists expressed it, he felt much as the captain of a 747 might have were he flying his aircraft with a hijacker's gun pointed at his head. Various strategies were discussed to bring the parents into closer touch with reality. One suggestion, later abandoned, was to require them to pay even a fraction of the cost of their baby's care— say one percent. (A number of recent studies have shown that where parents are even nominally responsible for the cost of their infant's care, decisions about withholding or withdrawing treatment tend to be made far more expeditiously than when the cost is being met by a third-party payer.) The next proposal was to insist that the parents spend a substantial amount of time, at least a week, in the nursery, participating in their child's care, instead of coming in briefly, once a month, proclaiming that all was well, and then going home.

The parents agreed to this latter request. After only three days at their infant's bedside, their attitude toward continued treatment underwent a complete reversal. They concurred with the view of the staff that their baby was not only failing to thrive, but was actually being ravaged by the well-intentioned interventions initially applied in the hope of saving his life. Very quickly, they consented to having their baby withdrawn from the breathing machine and medicated for pain. They held him as he died, hours later, finally at peace.

Parents Wanting Too Little Treatment

We have seen that parents sometimes want more done for their child than the team believes to be warranted on the basis of the available data. Not infrequently, the opposite problem is encountered: parents insisting that *less* be done for their baby than the team believes to be indicated by the evidence before them. The actual Baby Doe, of whom mention was made earlier, was a case in point. Most neonatologists and ancillary members of the intensive care team would place a Down's syndrome baby at that end of the spectrum where intensive care would obviously benefit the child. In this particular case, the parents were unwilling to accept anything less than a perfect baby. In many ways, this mind-set represents an unfortunate corollary of a liberal abortion law: since any defect is sufficient reason for a "therapeutic" abortion, why should genetic defects in babies actually born not provide similar grounds for decisions to let them die?

In the Baby Doe case, the treating physician simply went along with the parents' wishes, failing either to act in unilateral fashion as the baby's advocate or to consult with colleagues in order to make a medical decision based on accepted standards of treatment. The net result was federal intervention of the most unfortunate kind; it sought to circumscribe dramatically the discretion of physicians and parents in the decision-making process.

In institutions such as our own, the team will not hesitate to seek a court order to treat an infant whose parents want less done for her than seems to be medically indicated. Usually, a judge will provide such an order almost immediately, over the telephone. But what, it might be asked, if the parents then refuse to bear responsibility for any subsequent costs of treatment? On this point, too, courts have ruled. The liability remains theirs.

Both those parents who want more done for their child than seems to be medically appropriate and those who want less raise a more fundamental question about the nature of parenting. Does parenting mean ownership of a child, carrying with it the power to dispose over that infant's life or death? Or does it mean stewardship, caregiving— with the state appointing others to provide care for the child when the parents are unwilling or unable to do so themselves?

Surely, the latter rather than the former view of what it means to be parents must be upheld. None of us owns our children. At most, we are stewards entrusted with the responsibility of caring and providing for them. If we are unable or unwilling to do this, the state has the authority to step in and ensure that our children receive the care and provision to which they are entitled as members of the community. In the matter of medical care and provision, this means that the neonatal team occasionally may have to act as the instrument of society in assuring children the care to which they are entitled but which the parents are seeking to deny. Unfortunately, this can lead to an adversarial, rather than a collaborative, relationship with the parents involved. Yet when a life may be at stake, this is of less importance than acting decisively to save it.

Informed Consent

Another key ethical issue presented by the relationship between the parent or parents and the infant is that of informed consent. For most people who have not been exposed to it previously, the milieu of the neonatal intensive care unit represents a strange, confusing, and sometimes alarming new world. It is difficult to imagine a young couple entering such an environment with anything approaching confidence in their own autonomous decision-making power. When decisions must be made, they tend to be overly dependent on those providing care to their infant.

Yet it is the parents who must give consent for each fresh intervention on the part of the medical care team. Informed consent, at a minimum, requires substantial understanding of the problems confronting the child; of the available alternatives for dealing with these; and of the likely risks and benefits associated with each. It also demands substantial voluntariness: the couple being as uncoerced and as little manipulated as possible, so that their choices may be largely autonomous.

Such parents are typically in shock. They are mourning the loss of the normal, full-term baby they had expected; they are slowly coming to terms with the dread reality of what has actually happened to their baby and to them. Various studies have shown that people in shock simply do not hear what is said to them, even repeatedly, by those who endeavor to provide them with care. Obtaining an informed consent in such circumstances requires a reliable, repeated, and consistent feedback mechanism: "Please tell me what you think has been told you, and I will check your perceptions against what was actually said; if there is a gap between what was said and what you heard, we shall begin again, at the beginning. . . ."

In states like California, there may be ethnic, linguistic, and cultural barriers in the way of the parents providing a substantially informed and voluntary consent. At one neonatal intensive care center in the Stockton area, for example, there is a predominantly Vietnamese population. These parents of infants requiring intensive care typically understand little English. Additionally, there is a curious cultural difference between this ethnic group and those in the mainstream. According to Vietnamese tradition, it is the head of the clan, rather than the parents, who is invested with decision-making authority. The team typically attempts to engage the parents in the decision-making process. The parents in turn refer and defer to the head of the clan—whom the team does not have the opportunity to meet face to face, and who does not speak English at all. This makes communication convoluted and complicated in the extreme.

Finally, the fact that parents often live at some remove from the centers where their babies are receiving care raises further difficulties in the way of their informed participation. Neonatal intensive care centers tend to be regional; that is to say, they receive referrals from a large surrounding area. Inevitably, many parents will have long distances to travel to be with their babies and will not be able to stay with them for more than brief periods of time because of other pressing responsibilities at home. In such cases communication takes place predominantly over the telephone. The telephone is a notoriously inadequate instrument when it comes to obtaining a substantially informed and voluntary consent to complex and, from the parents' perspective, hitherto unheard-of procedures.

Overcoming these four obstacles requires considerable prowess and commitment on the part of the neonatal intensive care team. Social workers, translators, and chaplains of various religious persuasions render sterling service in facilitating communication, in lay language, between the neonatologists and the parents. Yet even with their help, informed consent remains problematic. None of us is ever certain that we have done more than a superficial job of involving parents in the difficult decisions associated with the care of their tiny babies. The ideal is ever before us. Attaining it always seems more elusive than we would like it to be.

Society Impinging on the Perinatal Team

As has been intimated, society, as represented minimally by third-party payers and the legal system, is steadily impinging on the perinatal team. Especially is this true now that we have entered an era of cost containment systems in the health care industry. This third corner of the triangle labeled "society," which formerly could conveniently be ignored by the providers of care, is moving uncomfortably close to the equilateral position. And this for good reason.

In an article quoted earlier, there is this brief but evocative paragraph:

> The mean length of stay among the survivors [in the 500–750-gram category of infants] was 137 days (range, 71 to 221), and the mean cost of care per infant was $158,800 (range, $72,110 to $524,110).[4]

Some commentators regard these figures as overly low. In any case, they require adjustment for inflation. Even without that, such statistics prompt the question: Is it morally justifiable to expend between $72,000 and $500,000 on an infant who has a 25 percent chance of surviving, and not more than a 70 percent prospect of surviving intact? The question becomes even more pointed when we consider what $72,000–$500,000 could do in terms of the prevention of prematurity.

Not only statisticians raise such a question; increasingly, it is being voiced by thoughtful commentators.[5] Common sense alone surely requires us to ask whether expending half a million dollars on an infant who dies after five months of heroic striving against the inevitable can possibly be justified when the same amount of money, invested in providing adequate prenatal care to indigent mothers-to-be, could preempt the need for such heroics in the first place, benefiting hundreds of children. Making this particular problem even more intractable is the fact that there is no real assurance that the $500,000 saved by not treating Baby A in a neonatal intensive care nursery would automatically benefit Babies B, C, D, E, F, and G *in utero* by providing their mothers with proper prenatal care. Cutting one slice of the pie smaller does not mean that other preferred pieces will inevitably become larger. In a society such as ours, with its special interest groups, the distribution of limited resources is not accomplished in such equitable and reasonable fashion!

Nevertheless, third-party payers might soon be asking, insistently and even stridently, whether the team can continue to be sanctioned to expend resources without regard to outcomes. Once this kind of questioning begins in earnest, the societal corner of the triangle will begin more and more to assert itself as to the way perinatal medicine is practiced. It could be that any failure now of the team to demonstrate restraint in terms of who is afforded intensive care will lead inexorably to constraints imposed later from without. Those who pay the piper surely have the right to call the tune. That they will exercise this right seems certain; it is merely a matter of time.

The societal corner of the triangle comprehends the law as well as economics. At present, there is little, if any, case law in the area of perinatology. In stark contrast, the practice of adult intensive care is now being informed by various far-reaching court decisions. Neither are there any neonatal equivalents of the various pieces of right-to-die legislation which have now become accepted in the adult arena. There are frequent appeals to judges for immediate rulings in particular cases where the team wants to provide the infants in their care with immediate treatments that the parents are unwilling to allow.

Unquestionably, this will also change with time. Wrongful birth and wrongful life suits loom on the horizon as the disabled begin to seek redress from those who made decisions which caused them to live, rather than allowing them to die. The litigiousness of our society is notorious. The pro-life lobby will not remain passive either; new strategies for mandating the treatment of all babies except those who are manifestly unsalvageable will be devised. Some of these will succeed and, in succeeding, will begin to regulate the practice of perinatology in unfortunate ways. And precedents in case law will emerge which will begin to affect the day-to-day decision-making process of the neonatal team in collaboration with parents—in direct and limiting fashion.

Months after I met her in the emergency department, I still wonder what became of Debbie, the "street person" to whom I ministered after the death of her premature baby. I collected about seven hundred dollars from friends to help her. Before she left the hospital, I had promised her I would do this and urged her to come back to see me and receive the money I felt sure I could solicit on her behalf. She never came. The money is in a fund used to help patients and family members down on their luck.

Even if she had come back, seven hundred dollars would have been but a drop in the bucket of her enormous need for drug rehabilitation, education, job training, employment, and affordable housing. Our society is doing little to meet such needs. One inevitable consequence is that women like Debbie give birth to premature, extremely-low-birthweight babies. We treat their babies in our neonatal intensive care units at extravagant cost. But we seem not to be able to treat their mothers with anything approaching compassion, respect, or justice.

Technology has a powerful fascination for us, as Americans. The vision of the civil rights years has dimmed somewhat, and we have begun to succumb to the myth that our society's unfortunates have only themselves to blame. So we invest resources in equipment and the buildings needed to house and deploy it but not in people. Investing in people would mean enabling the Debbies of our society to make a new, productive, and fulfilling life for themselves. It would mean providing them with adequate medical care while they are pregnant and affordable child care after their babies are born. It would mean practicing what the inscription on the Statue of Liberty proclaims. So long as we elect not to take these measures, the babies born to our Debbies will either die or else be rescued at incalculable financial and emotional cost. For in rescuing them, we may well succeed only in adding to the swelling numbers of totally dependent people in our midst. In the end, the choice—and its consequences—is ours alone.

9

Critical and
Terminal Care[1]

Jerry was 48 years old. He had amyotrophic lateral sclerosis—ALS, or
Lou Gehrig's disease, as it is commonly known. The disease is progressive and irreversible. It is characterized by a steady loss of muscle
and nerve function. Before the advent of breathing machines (ventilators),
victims of ALS died as soon as the muscles and nerves controlling respiration
were affected. Now it is possible to place these patients initially on portable,
then on hospital-based, ventilators, thereby extending their survival for some
years, albeit with a severely compromised quality of life.

Jerry's disease had progressed to the point where he could no longer breathe
without mechanical help. He had agreed to come into the hospital's intensive
care unit in order to assess what life on a ventilator was like. He had a
compact with his wife and two teenage children that if the experience of being
on a breathing machine compromised his own standards of independent
living, he would elect to die rather than continue in such fashion indefinitely.

His assessment of the experience, after two weeks on the ventilator, was
negative. Jerry communicated to his nurses and doctors his wish to be allowed
to die rather than be kept alive technologically. His wife realized that he was
adamant. Reluctantly, she agreed to abide by his decision. Together, they laid
out for the children the implications of Jerry's choice, and prepared them for
his eventual death.

However, before death could occur, Jerry's caregivers—his doctors and
nurses—had to agree that withdrawing ventilatory support was an ethically
appropriate as well as a legally prudent decision. I was invited to provide
the ethics consultation. After studying the facts of the case and talking with
him, I supported Jerry's request to be allowed to die naturally. He was clearly

conscious and competent, and therefore the principle of autonomy required all of us to accede to his wishes. Nevertheless, the legal ramifications for the hospital of Jerry's choice were potentially problematic. What if some family member later sued the hospital and its medical staff for not doing everything possible to keep their patient alive? The hospital's administrative represent- ative and legal counsel were called in to advise: how did they weigh Jerry's autonomous choice against the institution's need to be protected from mal- practice litigation? Within an impressively short space of time, Jerry's rela- tionship with his physicians had been expanded to include his family, his nurses, an ethics consultant, a hospital administrator, and hospital counsel.

More than death itself, most of us fear an inevitable process of dying meaninglessly and agonizingly protracted by artificial means in an alien environment. We are afraid that the instruments of healing will become the tools of torture; that the benefits of intensive care medicine will come to be outweighed by the harms inflicted in at- tempting to procure them. We want to believe that, for all of us, a time will arrive when death ought not any longer to be resisted and fought back as an enemy, by any and all means possible, but instead might be welcomed and embraced as a friend. We are fearful that this moment would not be recognized by those on whom we, or our loved ones, might well become dependent for medical care were we or they to become critically or terminally ill. Our technological ability to pre- serve and extend life, especially in intensive care units, more often than not commands admiration. For a minority of patients, however, those whose physical existence can be extended only at the price of prolonging their dying, the technology of the intensive care unit has acquired more sinister and dread connotations.

To Prolong Life or to End Suffering?

Sometimes it seems that an overwhelming fascination, even in- fatuation, with the toys of technology prompts intensivists un- concernedly to play with them, even in circumstances too se- rious for mere games. Besides, intensivists, like other physicians, are often genuinely concerned that if they do not do everything possible for their patients, unquestioningly and unremittingly, they will later be sued. The defensive and overly conservative practice of medicine is an inevitable corollary to the litigiousness of American society.

Fortunately, there are now some good legal precedents for at times not doing everything it is possible to do. Also, the American Medical and Bar associations are beginning to search for alternatives to malpractice litigation to compensate and redress aggrieved consumers. These negotiations, however, are still in their early stages. The threat of malpractice litigation remains anything but vague.

Intensivists sometimes miss seeing the line between extending life and prolonging death because those involved in the decision making process are many and speak with various voices. In the intensive care unit of a modern medical center, the responsibility of ethical decision-making may extend beyond the patient and the primary community physician to include the family, the director of the intensive care unit and her associates, the medical house staff, the nurses, the respiratory therapists, the social worker, the chaplain, the ethics consultant or committee, and the hospital's legal counsel! This complicates matters extraordinarily. Far simpler not to make any decision at all than to strive for an ethical consensus among such a disparate group. Yet not to decide is itself a decision. And in the arena of critical and terminal care, it is one that can have momentous consequences for patients and families.

Beneficence vs. Nonmaleficence

As we have seen, two primary medico-moral principles serve to guide the practice of medicine: *beneficence,* which requires the attempt to preserve life, and *nonmaleficence,* which mandates the alleviation of suffering. Usually the two primary principles can be applied concurrently, without conflict, to inform the physician's decisions. In circumstances of critical or terminal illness, however, they sometimes come into conflict. Then it becomes possible to apply one principle only at the expense of the other: to preserve life may inflict rather than alleviate suffering; to alleviate suffering may require abandoning the intention to continue to preserve life. In such situations, where principles are in opposition to one another, one might well ask, "Which ought to take precedence over the other, and when, and why?"

There are those who adroitly resolve a conflict between the two traditional medico-moral principles by simply insisting that always and in all circumstances preserving life ought to take precedence over the concern to alleviate suffering. In terms of Figure 9-1, if X represents birth, Y death, and the curve the human lifespan, they insist that from X through Y care ought to take the form of an unyielding and unremitting attempt to cure. That is to say, the sanctity of the patient's life is valued above its quality, and death is perceived as an enemy to be fought back and kept at bay by every means for as long as possible.

Patients as well as physicians may espouse this absolutistic philosophy of care for a variety of reasons. Some patients may have urgent, unfinished business to attend to before they die: the writing of a symphony to complete, a financial transaction to finalize, a legacy of one kind or another to ensure. Understandably, they might be willing to purchase whatever time they can, without regard for the quality of their lives, by insisting that everything possible be done to maintain their physical existence.

Others, quite simply, might be unable to come to terms with their own mortality. The threat of non-being is so intense that they would be willing to endure all kinds of harm, whether iatrogenic (physician induced) or disease-related in order to hold at bay the inevitable. I suspect that many in this category support the cryonics fad of storing bodies in liquid nitrogen against the day when cures will have been discovered for the diseases which caused death, when the bodies will be warmed up, the treatments applied, and immortality gained. Such claims on the part of the cryonics industry are patently unscientific and spurious.

Figure 9-1: Schematic Representation of the Life Cycle

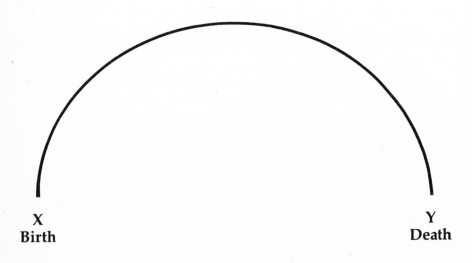

X
Birth

Y
Death

Various motives may lurk behind the adoption by physicians of a philosophy in which care is equated with the unswerving attempt to cure. One has to do with research. If a dramatic breakthrough can be achieved in treating a patient with what in the present state of knowledge is regarded as an incurable and terminal condition, this may benefit a whole population of those similarly affected. Another motive may be at work in cases where the patients are children with terminal disease.

For children afflicted with terminal illnesses, research will often be an overriding consideration: an extra year or two, purchased at no matter what price, would represent a major proportion of the lifespan of a 7- or 9-year-old; it would be a much less significant fraction of the lifespan of a 70- or 90-year-old. Additionally, there might be a further justification for thinking of care only in terms of the attempt to cure: just as there are patients temperamentally incapable of coming to terms with their inevitable finitude, so there are physicians unable to accept defeat. Unfortunately, to stop treating a terminal disease aggressively is, for many, tantamount to admitting defeat.

There is, however, another way of looking at this configuration, of conceptualizing what it means to care responsibly and humanely. It

Figure 9-2: Alternative Conceptualizations of What it Means to Care

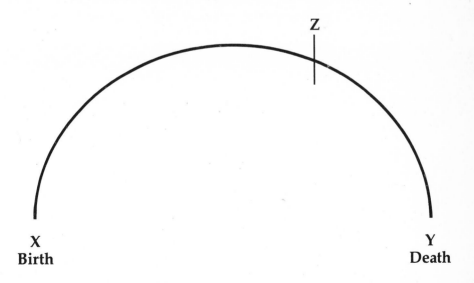

is posited on the basis of point Z in Figure 9-2. Point Z may be defined as the moment when the difference is recognized between attempting to extend life with meaning, as defined by the patient herself, and prolonging an inevitable process of dying in mindless and meaningless fashion. To be sure, discerning point Z is difficult. Three factors, at least, enter into the process of determining that this point has arrived.

One is the acquisition of objective clinical data: X-rays, magnetic resonance imaging (MRI), or computerized tomography (CT) scanning indicating that the disease is not being contained, further findings of untreatable metastases, disastrous blood counts, etc. A second is the subjective assessment of the patient himself that, having striven valiantly against the disease, the fight is no longer worth the candle. So far as the patient is concerned, the deleterious consequences of continuing the struggle far outweigh the benefit of sheer survival without discernible quality. And, third, there is intuition: the intuition of either the clinician or the patient, or both, that the time has come to move from a strategy in which attempting to extend life has been the paramount concern to a view in which the quality of life must now be seen as more important—when, finally, death may be welcomed.

If it is conceded that determining point Z on the X-Y curve is possible (and, obviously, doing this will perhaps require more in terms of the art of medicine than its science), then another philosophy of care suggests itself. From X through Z, the principle of preserving life ought to take precedence over that of alleviating suffering; the value of the sanctity of life ought to predominate over quality-of-life considerations; death ought to be seen more as an enemy to be kept at bay than as a welcome visitant; and care ought to take the form of the resolute attempt to cure.

But from Z through Y, the ranking of these principles and values may be reversed. Now alleviating suffering may and ought to take precedence over the principle of attempting to preserve life. Now the quality of life may receive more emphasis than the mere prolongation of physical existence. Now death may appropriately be recognized as a friend to be embraced. Now care may take the form of ensuring comfort in the face of pain, affording constant companionship to the dying person rather than abandoning or isolating her—much easier in a home or hospice setting than in a hospital—and facilitating a creative completion of the patient's inner journey, which will move spiritual counselors and ministrants from the wings to center stage. And now it will also be possible to regard the withdrawal or withholding of aggressive life-sustaining technologies as an appropriate expression of care.

Ethical Guidelines in Intensive Care Units

Of those who are patients in intensive care units, some will inevitably come to be diagnosed as terminally ill; their disease process will be seen as irreversible. Let us look at the range of principles that facilitate decision making about the withdrawal or withholding of aggressive, heroic, life-sustaining technologies in such cases, and identify the principals potentially party to the decision making process, along with their appropriate roles.

There are some guidelines to help the intensivist in making complex ethical decisions. We shall examine five that serve as broad principles, rather than as rigid and inflexible rules.

The first is a common-sense criterion. It is that the standard for admission to and continuance in an intensive care unit be the potential for salvageability. Cynthia Cohen, a commentator on the ethics of intensive care, states it thus:

> All who are critically ill should not automatically be admitted to the ICU. A necessary condition for admission is that the patient be potentially salvageable, by which it is meant that the patient has a chance for returning to a state in which his or her life is not threatened. Patients who are immediately and irreversibly dying, and for whom it has been carefully determined that there is no known therapy, are not salvageable. They deserve comfort and support within the hospital but cannot benefit from intensive care.[2]

With respect to this standard, two qualifications are necessary: first, that it is easier to apply at the time of admission to an ICU than when the de-escalation of intensive care technology is being contemplated because a patient is no longer thought to be salvageable. At the outset, when admission to an ICU is an option, that the patient be believed to have a slim (10 percent to 40 percent) chance of recovery is usually sufficient to justify an aggressive attempt to preserve his life. When it becomes apparent, however, that the patient is no longer salvageable and that comfort and support are more appropriate than intensive care, a far higher level of certainty is required. Before agreeing to the withholding or withdrawal of life-sustaining therapies because of the belief that the patient is at point Z, the intensivist reaches for a degree of certainty approaching 100 percent, rather than the considerably lower level that sufficed at the beginning.

A second variable affecting the guideline is that the definition of salvageability is largely determined by the available resources. A simple analogy may serve to make this point. If one were fortunate enough to inherit a Model A Ford and wanted it restored to its pristine condition, there are craftsmen who can do this. Their work is beautiful to behold. So long as there were no limit to the funds one was willing to expend on such an enterprise, it is entirely possible that the Ford could be fully restored, with genuine parts, or with parts hand-made to the original specifications. However, if one had to work within a restricted budget of, let us say, $5,000, it is highly unlikely that the same goal could be attained. For $5,000 it might be possible to restore the upholstery or the chassis or the motor, or even the body to mint condition. But it is too much to hope that the whole car could be renovated. Labor and parts together would carry the cost beyond the $5,000 available.

So long as resources are infinite, or are believed to be infinite, as was the case when intensive care units began to proliferate in the 1960s, the definition of salvageability can be loose, and the threshold for admittance to and continuance in an intensive care unit can be low. Once it is recognized that resources are finite and that limits on expenditures have to be set, as is now the case within cost-containment systems of reimbursement, the definition of salvageability necessarily becomes more stringent. At the same time, the threshold of eligibility for intensive care may have to be raised.

These two qualifications notwithstanding, the salvageability criterion is a useful one. It reminds us that caring can encompass several different activities. At times, caring may require cardiopulmonary resuscitation, respirators, powerful drugs, renal dialysis, or other such invasive measures. On other occasions, it warrants no more than palliation for pain and the discomfort, for example, of constipation or bedsores. It is to be hoped that caring never ceases. However, the form caring takes will be dictated by medical and other factors.

This guideline accords well with the conclusions of a Consensus Development Conference, recently held at the National Institutes of

Health, to discuss issues related to the practice of critical care medicine. Speakers at the conference identified three categories of patients:

- those "with acute reversible disease for whom the probability of survival without ICU intervention is low, but the survival probability with such intervention is high";

- those "with a low probability of survival without intensive care whose probability of survival with intensive care may be higher—but the potential benefit is not as clear";

- those "admitted to the ICU, not because they are critically ill, but because they are at risk of becoming critically ill. The purpose of intensive care in these instances [is] to prevent a serious complication or to allow a prompt response to any complication that may occur."

The report went on to state that

it is not medically appropriate to devote limited ICU resources to patients without reasonable prospect of significant recovery when patients who need those services and who have a significant prospect of recovery from acutely life-threatening disease or injury are being turned away due to a lack of capacity. It is inappropriate to maintain ICU management of a patient whose prognosis has resolved to one of persistent vegetative state, and it is similarly inappropriate to employ ICU resources where no purpose will be served but a prolongation of the natural processes of death.[3]

Traditional Principles

Beneficence imposes on the physician the duty of attempting to preserve life. It is the driving force behind critical care medicine. The impressive technological accomplishments commonplace in modern intensive care units all stem from this primary medico-moral imperative. The principle of nonmaleficence, a duty at least not to harm the patient, even if she cannot be benefited, is also incumbent on the physician.

Unfortunately, the environment of an intensive care unit is itself potentially harmful, if not lethal. This may seem to be a paradoxical assertion. Are not ICUs designed to benefit those who are seriously or critically ill? How can they possibly be harmful, in and of themselves? The reason is close at hand: because of their inactivity and their being kept typically in the prone position, patients in intensive care units are susceptible to many kinds of infections, particularly of the lungs. Antibiotic drugs are used to fight these infections. However, the microorganisms responsible for the infections are diabolically clever. They mutate and in mutating become resistant to the drugs that formerly would have destroyed them. In their mutated state they are prevalent within the ICU environment.

The mutated microorganisms might be thought of as predators with a natural prey—the intensive care unit patient. Therefore, as a general rule, it is true to say that whereas intensive care can benefit patients, providing they are in and out within a few days, the longer one is in an intensive care setting, the greater is the likelihood of one's being harmed by iatrogenic (physician-induced) factors.

Nonmaleficence, the duty not to harm, entails, as a corollary, a concern to alleviate suffering, whether physical or psychological. For the most part, in medicine, it is possible to apply the first principle, that of endeavoring to preserve life, and this second principle, doing no harm or alleviating suffering, concurrently and without conflict. As we have seen, however, in circumstances of terminal illness, the one principle can usually be upheld only at the expense of the other. Then a choice has to be made about which principle should predominate, and when, and why. We will return to this point.

Additionally, there is the principle of *autonomy*. This principle, rooted in the Judeo-Christian tradition, blossomed during the Renaissance through the writings of such people as Immanuel Kant and, as we have seen, has come to fruition in our own culture and in our own time. The net effect has been to make the patient central to the decision-making process. It is now axiomatic that no decision should be arrived at about patients' treatment or non-treatment, without their, or their designated proxies, having been consulted.

Finally, there is the principle of *justice*.[4] The principle of distributive justice, or fairness, often invoked in an era of cost-containment systems, presses upon us the questions: How can we fairly allocate expensive intensive care unit resources? How can we equitably distribute among the many claimants for our services those relatively limited benefits we have to offer? Although it is not the purpose of this chapter to explore answers that have been, and might be, proposed, the questions are always in the background while the drama of intensive care is being enacted. Today, the economics of health care cannot be divorced from the ethics of health care.

One point, however, about which I feel strongly is that decisions within the ICU ought never to be made on economic, rather than on medical, grounds. From an ethical point of view, it is simply not acceptable to decide to discontinue aggressive therapy because it is thought to be costing too much. To do this would be to violate the moral agreement implicitly entered into with the patient at the time of admission. (This position was independently endorsed by the National Institutes of Health Consensus Development Conference on Critical Care Medicine.)

It is nevertheless morally acceptable for considerations of cost, dictated by the principle of distributive justice, to enter into the decision-making process before the patient is admitted to the ICU. Given the relative limits of our present-day resources, for a hospital to decide not to afford intensive care, for example, to any patient with an underlying metastatic, terminal disease process would be morally acceptable. So long as this policy was declared beforehand to staff members and patients and their family members, there could be no moral objection to an administrative decision to be more selective in admitting patients to the ICU.

These basic ethical principles pertinent to decision making in the intensive care unit are always in tension and sometimes in conflict with one another. For example, the tension between beneficence and nonmaleficence is expressed in terms of a risk-benefit ratio; that between beneficence and justice through a cost-benefit assessment. Autonomy may prompt me to ask for more in the way of costly treatments than is medically indicated; distributive justice may require my autonomy to be circumscribed to some degree. Therefore, a rationale for ranking these guidelines in order of priority when they do conflict with one another must be proposed.

Ranking Conflicting Principles

What was said earlier bears repeating here. So long as the patient is still considered to be salvageable, the goal of preserving life, *beneficence*, ought to take precedence over the principle of doing no harm or alleviating suffering, *nonmaleficence*. However, once it has been determined that a patient is no longer salvageable, intensive care is not the most appropriate form of care, and the principle of nonmaleficence assumes priority over benefi-

Table 9-1: Principals Potentially Party

	Interest in the Decision-Making Process	Obstacles in the Way of Doing This
The Patient Should, ideally, play the *primary* and *central* role in limiting therapy.	Not wanting death prolonged when life cannot be further extended with meaning and quality according to the patient's own definition. *Principle:* Autonomy	None, so long as the patient is conscious and competent *and* "unsalvageable" (irreversibly terminal).
		Unconsciousness or incompetence
		The patient not yet seen as "unsalvageable," the disease process not yet seen as irreversible and terminal.
The Family Should, ideally, play a role *secondary* to the patient and *advisory* to the team in decisions to limit therapy.	(i) Same as the patient's, expressed above *Principle:* As above	The family's guilt over "ending the patient's life" by their decision. Defining "quality" of life for someone else.
	(ii) Wanting to end their own suffering, rather than the patient's.	The team's contract is always with the patient first and foremost; the family is secondary.
	(iii) Ulterior motivation: wanting to save further expense, or the desire to inherit.	Again, the patient's interests take precedence over those of the family. Decisions must be made on medical, not economic grounds.
The Critical Care Team Should, ideally, play a role *secondary* to the patient, but more *assertive* than the family in limiting therapy.	Medical judgment about "unsalvageability" with the patient now perceived as terminal.	Unrealistic attitudes in the family. Family members with unfinished business to complete. Legal hazards of withdrawing ventilatory, then intravenous, support. The case of *Clarence Herbert*.
	Medical judgment about the irreversibility of the patient's condition (vegetative state).	
The Hospital as an Institution	Fear of malpractice litigation may cause dying to be prolonged. Concern to conserve shrinking DRG resources may cause living not to be extended.	Institutional intrusion into the privacy of the physician-patient relationship, now an inevitability; conflict with patient autonomy.
Society *Economically:* Society should *not* make decisions within the ICU itself.	*Principles:* Nonmaleficence, alleviating suffering	Policy decisions are typically made in *ad hoc* fashion, not in rational, principled manner.
	Conservation of scarce resources *Principle:* Distributive Justice	
Legally: Court decisions affect what happens in the ICU; as do state and federal legislation.	Autonomy of the patient	Varies from state to state
	Assisted Suicide	Right-to-Life lobby

to the Decision-Making Process

How These Obstacles May Be Overcome	Remaining Problems
Appeal to the "right to refuse treatment," recognized by the AMA and the AHA.	The case of *Mr. Bartling*
Natural Death Act (or its equivalent). Durable Power of Attorney for Health Care.	Ignorance or neglect of these measures. Patient not legally "qualified." Patient not identified as having executed such a document.
Either: The Bartling precedent Or: The team continuing to treat. For how long? The case of *Elizabeth Bouvia*.	Risk of litigation for assault and battery or negligence.
Prior unambiguous, regularly updated written statements of patient's wishes. Verbal testimony.	Absence of any such statement, written or verbal. The family divided in its opinions.
The team continuing to act in accordance with the *patient's* expressed wishes (if known), or according to the *patient's* best interest, medically perceived.	The possibility of legal repercussions from disgruntled family members. Documenting all decisions and collaborative decision-making important.
Continuing treatment *and* initiating emotional and spiritual support of family until family ready to let go. AMA guidelines following the *Barber* case.	The possibility of civil, but not criminal, legal repercussions.
New Jersey Supreme Court ruling in the cases of *Hilda Peter, Nancy Jobes,* and *Kathleen Farrell* (June, 1987).	The need for more legislative guidelines.
Institutional guidelines for eligibility for ICU services, publicly proclaimed. Societal involvement in policy decisions.	The increased bureaucratization of medicine. Policies applicable across the board do not sufficiently allow for the uniqueness of individuals.
Lobbying for National Standards	What is ethical is being reduced to what is legal.
Education, lobbying	

cence. Defining salvageability, both medically and in terms of the resources available, is the key to reranking principles and reordering priorities from curing to comforting.

Autonomy ought to have its place throughout the decision-making process. As far as possible, medical decisions ought never to be made by physicians acting unilaterally. To involve patients in the decision-making process, thus respecting and upholding their autonomy, is usually not difficult, so long as they continue to be conscious and competent. The exercise of patient autonomy becomes problematic only when patients are unconscious or incompetent, as is often the case in the emergency room setting. Various attempts have been made to meet this difficulty, extending autonomy beyond the point when the patient is no longer conscious or competent. These will be mentioned later.

The final principle, *distributive justice*, ought to have its place outside the ICU, in the area of institutional and public policy, rather than within the intensive care unit itself. Once having initiated treatment for medical reasons, it is simply unacceptable to terminate treatment on economic grounds. Economic considerations do, however, have a legitimate place in deciding which patients not to treat intensively when first admitted. Physicians as well as patients need to come to terms with the fact that medicine is simply unable to postpone death indefinitely.

When it has become apparent that the patient is no longer salvageable, doing no harm—or alleviating suffering—will become more important than continuing with the futile and potentially harmful attempt to preserve life. Once intensive care is seen to be no longer the most appropriate form of care, and palliative or supportive care is indicated, who can and who ought to decide to limit treatment? Who are the principals who might apply the principles we have been discussing? A summary answer to this question is provided in Table 9-1.

From Principles to Principals

The Patient

The principle of autonomy requires that patients assume the primary role in all decisions to limit therapy, whenever this can be managed. Typically, the patient's interest in deciding to limit therapy is that of not wanting the process of dying to be meaninglessly and painfully prolonged when life can no longer be extended with quality, according to his or her own definition. Patients in this category present an unusual ethical problem: to what extent does an unsalvageable patient have the right to command costly and increasingly scarce intensive care unit resources in a futile attempt to hold death at bay? In such a case, the principles of autonomy and justice collide. Since autonomy is never an absolute, this may well be an instance where society's concern for the common good, grounded in the principle of justice, may have to take precedence over the principle of autonomy, inadequately construed as unbridled freedom.

So long as the patient is conscious and competent, there are no insurmountable obstacles in the way of his exercising the right to refuse treatment. This right has been recognized both by the American Medical Association and by the American Hospital Association, and is included in the widely available Patient's Bill of Rights. The case of *Bartling v. Superior Court*,[5] however, is a reminder that this right cannot be taken for granted and that it has now been upheld by court action in a single jurisdiction. Mr. Bartling, 70 years old, had multiple medical problems. His condition had become compromised after a pneumothorax sustained during a biopsy of a lung mass. He had a chest tube inserted, was tracheotomized, and was placed on a respirator.

Throughout his hospital stay, Mr. Bartling remained conscious and competent. On several occasions, he attempted to remove the respirator tubes, and he repeatedly requested that ventilatory support be discontinued. The treating physicians and the hospital refused to do this and continued to restrain Mr. Bartling so that he could not extubate himself. Richard S. Scott, a doctor and lawyer active in the right-to-die movement, took up this case on Mr. Bartling's behalf. The lower court denied Scott's request for an injunction restraining the hospital and the physicians from administering medical care to which the patient had not given consent. The case was appealed. Before the appeal court had adjudicated, Mr. Bartling died, still connected to his ventilator. However, so important was this case deemed to be that a higher court ruled posthumously, holding that

> competent adult patients, with serious illnesses which are probably incurable, but have not been diagnosed as terminal, have the right, over the objection of their physicians and the hospital, to have life-support equipment discon-

nected despite the fact that withdrawal of such devices will surely hasten death.

Usually, obstacles in the way of patients limiting intensive care therapy arise only when they become either unconscious or incompetent. In the context of the ICU, incompetency has a narrow definition; it simply means that one is adjudged to be incapable of making a rational medical decision affecting one's own person. From the patient's point of view, a paramount concern is, "How can I continue to exercise my autonomy when I become unconscious or incompetent?" And from the physician's perspective, an equally important consideration is, "How do I carry out what seem to be the patient's wishes, without becoming overly vulnerable to malpractice litigation?"

Early attempts to address these issues included the so-called Living Will (never recognized as a legally valid document) and the California Natural Death Act, or its equivalent. California's statute had several deficiencies. One major problem was that, according to the provisions of the act, its directive to physicians could be executed only by persons who were at the time, and had been for at least fourteen days previously, terminally ill—as defined in the act itself. Mr. Bartling was not terminally ill, according to this definition, when he asked to be allowed to exercise his right to refuse treatment. This prevents its being of assistance to those who, not being terminally ill beforehand, go on later to sustain massive, irreversible neurological or physiological damage, or both, whether accidentally or iatrogenically, and whose relatives and caregivers want to allow them to die naturally.

Because of these difficulties, California later legislated its "proxy directive," commonly known as The Durable Power of Attorney for Health Care, in January, 1985. This document empowers any other person selected by the patient to make decisions regarding health care on the patient's behalf and in accordance with his or her expressed wishes, if he or she should later become unconscious or incompetent. Ordinary powers of attorney do not survive their makers' incompetence. This one, however, remains in effect—hence its designation, "durable." Several other states have enacted similar legislation. All give expression to a recommendation of a presidential commission that durable powers of attorney be preferred to living wills, "since they are more generally applicable and provide a better vehicle for patients to exercise self-determination."[6]

Attending physicians frequently have difficulty in simply acceding to a patient's request to terminate life-sustaining treatment when the patient is not yet deemed to be unsalvageable or terminal on medical grounds. For a salvageable or nonterminal patient to refuse treatment that could possibly restore her to functionality, at least for the foreseeable future, seems tantamount to a suicidal death wish or evidence of insanity. The beneficent, albeit paternalistic, impulse in such cases is to continue treating, hoping that either the suicidal desire or the incompetency will prove temporary and will later yield to retrospective consent to the treatments given.

Yet there are people like Mr. Bartling in intensive care units who are neither terminal, nor crazy, nor irrationally suicidal. Competently and thoughtfully, they wish to exercise their right not to receive further aggressive therapy. Attending physicians are then wedged in a predicament: either to honor the patient's wishes at the risk of being sued later by some distant family member or to overrule patient autonomy in order to protect their own interests. Either way, there are risks. Ethics and the law may lead in different directions. From the point of view of ethics, a patient's wishes, however unacceptable, must never be discounted—so long as they are authentically autonomous. In light of possible legal repercussions, however, physicians in such situations may deem it prudent to continue to attempt to preserve the patient's life.

The Family

If the principle of patient autonomy is to be taken seriously, the role of the family in decisions to limit therapy should be secondary to that of the patient. The family's function should be advisory to the critical care team rather than assertive—an important distinction. To shift the authority for decision-making from the critical care team to the family when the patient can no longer be actively involved in the decision making process would, concomitantly, saddle relatives with responsibility for the decision arrived at. This could cause them to feel guilty about decisions resulting in the death of the patient.

Since it is the underlying disease process that usually causes patients to die, not the withdrawal or withholding of life-sustaining measures, it seems unnecessarily cruel to saddle the family with a burden of guilt for the decision to limit futile intensive care. It is preferable for the critical care team to consult closely with the family in order to act in accordance with their interpretation of the patient's wishes, yet to assume responsibility themselves for the decisions eventually made.

In an ideal situation, the family's interest in limiting therapy would be identical to that of the patient: not wanting dying to be protracted when life, characterized by capacities consistent with the patient's own self-understanding and definition of quality of life, cannot any longer be extended. In such cases, the assumption is that the family knows what capabilities the patient would have considered indispensable for a meaningful life.

Where there is good reason to believe that the family genuinely and unanimously represents the patient's wishes and interests, either because of a prior written statement, or a signed legal document, or the patient's reiterated verbal communications, few difficulties can be imagined. But in situations where there was no written or verbal statement by the patient beforehand and, to make matters worse, where the family is divided in its opinions about what the patient would have wanted, the conclusion is inescapable that the critical care team has no alternative but to proceed conservatively, continuing the treatment regimen. In medicine, as in life, discretion is occasionally the better part of valor.

Sometimes the critical care team may have reason to suspect that the family is not representing the patient's best interests but is advancing their own instead. For example, the team may have a hunch that the family is seeking to alleviate their own suffering rather than that of the patient or, worse, is eager to hasten the patient's demise in order to inherit an estate. Whenever such speculations seem well founded, the members of the team have little alternative, morally speaking, but to remind themselves that their primary obligation is to the patient, not to the family, even though the family may be the legal surrogate decision maker. In such an event, the team will continue to act either in accordance with the patient's expressed wishes or in what they consider the patient's best interests, medically perceived. The reasons for following this course should be carefully documented in the patient's chart; there is always the possibility that disaffected family members will later initiate malpractice litigation.

The Critical Care Team

What makes modern intensive care possible at all, apart from technology, is the sophistication and concentration of intensive care nurses in such units. It is they, not the machines, who provide intensive care.

Because of their extensive technical, pharmacological, psychological, and nursing expertise, registered nurses have claimed and are steadily asserting their own distinct professional identity. No longer are they willing to be subservient to physicians; they are acknowledged caregivers in their own right and insist on being recognized as such. Nurses have a pivotal role to play in the communication process: between other members of the team, between the team and the patient and family, and between various family members. For these reasons, it is important that nurses in intensive care units be regarded as colleagues by physicians and be accorded their due place on the team, especially with respect to the process of making decisions about the withholding or withdrawal of intensive care therapies.

Other members of the team may include community physicians, house officers in teaching hospitals, respiratory therapists, social workers, chaplains, and—more and more—an ethics consultant or hospital ethics committee representative. Tension between members of the team sparked by disagreement about the moral and medical propriety of some decisions is inevitable. A recent article in the *Journal of the American Medical Association* draws attention to the fact that medical residents at the bedside frequently feel that the attending physicians are out of touch with current problems and ethical approaches. Residents experience considerable stress when those to whom they are responsible fail to discuss their decisions with them beforehand yet expect unquestioning compliance. This prompts the observation that

> little attention has been paid to the issue of whether residents are always bound to the decisions of their attending physicians, and whether it may ever be appropriate for residents to decline to participate in the life-sustaining care of patients on the basis of ethical grounds.[7]

Although the attending ICU physicians bear ultimate responsibility for decisions made in the ICU, those that are complex should be arrived at collaboratively rather than unilaterally. This not only makes good sense in terms of human interactions and relationships within the unit but also is prudent, given the litigiousness of our society. A decision, however controversial, that has been thoroughly discussed among the members of the team, carefully arrived at, and meticulously documented is the best means of alleviating the fear of subsequent litigation.

The team's role in limiting therapy should be secondary to that of the patient—again, because of the principle of autonomy—but assertive, not merely advisory. Physicians, not family members per se, are licensed to practice medicine. Assertiveness on the part of the team after careful consultation with the family can reduce the family's guilt over "deciding to end the patient's life" by reminding them that it is the disease or the accident that brought the patient to the ICU which will ultimately end his or her life, rather than a decision to end meaningless suffering.

The interest of the team in deciding to limit therapy ought to be primarily medical, with regard to a patient's unsalvageability or the irreversible nature of a patient's condition. Such determinations trigger the substitution of one form of care (palliative) for another (intensive), with the attempt to assure the patient's comfort supplanting the heroic attempt to cure. The principle of alleviating suffering now predominates over the principle of preserving life, and death may be anticipated as a welcome release.

Implementing decisions arrived at in this way may be delayed for humanitarian reasons and resisted for fear of legal repercussions. The humanitarian concerns could include allowing a family with an unrealistic view of the patient's condition the time they will need to adjust to what the prognosis really is, or affording members of the family the opportunity to complete any unfinished business with the patient. The following anecdote illustrates this last point:

After a 51-year-old patient in our ICU had been determined to be legally brain dead, she was ventilated for another week to allow her 18-year-old son time to complete his own unfinished business with her. He had left home angrily a year earlier and had not seen his mother since. His siblings were present with her before her surgery (from which she never recovered), but he was not. When he eventually arrived at the hospital, his mother was unresponsive. Nevertheless, he was encouraged to talk to her as if she could hear and understand what was being said. During the week before ventilatory support was discontinued, he told her that he was sorry about his earlier behavior and that he loved her. Finally, when he had expressed what he had not previously been able to say and had begun to forgive himself for what had been amiss in his relationship with his mother, respiratory support was discontinued. The patient died immediately.

Physicians

Fear of legal repercussions has been the major reason for hesitancy to execute decisions based on good medical grounds. Initially, this fear was exacerbated by the case of *People v. Barber*[8], in which two physicians, Leonard Barber and Robert Nejdl, were charged with murder and conspiracy to commit murder after life-sustaining measures were withdrawn from Clarence Herbert, a patient in a deeply comatose state, in accordance with the wishes of his family.

Clarence Herbert, a 55-year-old security guard, had come into the hospital for an ileostomy closure. The operation had been completed successfully. While in the recovery room, Mr. Herbert went into cardiopulmonary arrest. He was resuscitated, intubated, and transported to the ICU, where he was placed on a respirator. He was never again to regain consciousness. He went into what the physicians described as an irreversible coma, secondary to extensive brain damage. The electroencephalogram (EEG) showed minimal brain activity. Mrs. Herbert and her eight children unanimously asked that ventilatory support be withdrawn from Clarence Herbert, and that he be allowed to die naturally. They went so far as to express this in writing: "We, the immediate family of Clarence LeRoy Herbert, would like all machines taken off that are sustaining life. We release all liability to Hosp. Dr. & Staff."

Three days after his cardiopulmonary arrest, the patient was removed from the breathing machine. To the dismay of all concerned, Mr. Herbert did not die; he continued breathing spontaneously. Two days later, at the family's insistence that intravenous lines providing hydration be withdrawn and that the nasogastric feeding tube be removed in compliance with their written request that "all machines [be] taken off that are sustaining life," Mr. Herbert ceased to receive hydration and nourishment. Six days later, he died.

Sandra Bardenilla, an ICU nurse, called the county health services department to file a formal complaint; the department referred the case to the district attorney. Deputy District Attorney Nikola M. Mikulicich initiated the prosecution of Drs. Barber and Nejdl for murder. The physicians petitioned the court of appeal to issue a writ of prohibition against the trial court, restraining it from taking further action against them. The court of appeal did so, with Justice Fleming observing that "a murder prosecution is a poor way to design an ethical and moral code for doctors who are faced with decisions concerning the use of costly and extraordinary 'life support' equipment."[9]

Although the criminal charges against Drs. Barber and Nejdl were dismissed, they still face a civil action. Mrs. Herbert has been prevailed upon to sue for malpractice. This issue has not yet been settled.

Based on the decision in *Barber v. Superior Court*, the Board of the Los Angeles County Bar Association approved, on December 11, 1985, and the Board of the Los Angeles County Medical Association ratified, on January 6, 1986, a document entitled "Principles and Guidelines Concerning the Foregoing of Life-Sustaining Treatment for Adult Patients." In this document, it is expressly stated that

> all life-sustaining interventions, including nutrition and hydration, are legally equivalent. It is legally acceptable for the caregiver to withhold or withdraw any or all of them. It is recognized, however, that nutrition and hydration have a powerful symbolic significance to both the members of the general public and to many caregivers.

This means that the insertion of intravenous lines and nasogastric feeding tubes has come to be regarded as medical intervention, not as a basic requirement.

In March of 1986, the American Medical Association's judicial council approved a new policy on withdrawing medical treatment. In this far-reaching policy statement, the AMA proclaims that it would be ethical for doctors to withhold "all means of life-prolonging medical treatment, including food and water, from patients in irreversible comas." The court decision in *People v. Barber*, these two policy statements by the joint committee of the Los Angeles County Bar and Medical associations on biomedical ethics, and the position now adopted by the American Medical Association should go a long way toward alleviating intensivists' fears that the withdrawal or withholding of life-sustaining interventions, including hydration and nutrition by means of IV and NG feeding tubes, respectively, could result in criminal action against them. However, the possibility of civil action remains, as the continuing ordeal of Leonard Barber and Robert Nejdl attests.

Hospitals

In recent years, the hospital as an institution has tended to intrude, more and more, into decisions about limiting therapy. Although the decision-making prerogative properly belongs to the patient, in collaboration with the treating physicians, the hospital can be motivated to usurp it for at least two reasons, both having to do with economics. First, the hospital may be concerned that malpractice litigation would reflect adversely on the institution. Were it not for the fact that these are days of stringent financial constraints, this eventuality would not loom large. After all, it is not the hospital so much as its insurer that bears the brunt of those legal claims that are upheld. However, the adverse publicity associated with successful malpractice suits could cost the hospital patients—and, therefore, revenue.

The hospital industry has become highly competitive. Marketing strategies and public relations endeavors are designed to woo and win patients for one hospital from others in the same geographical area. It is this concern that has caused administrators to become involved in the decision-making process. One of their overriding interests is to avert negative publicity that will reflect poorly on the institution.

Coupled with this is a converse but, it is to be hoped, less likely possibility: hospital administrators not wanting patients with limited or no financial coverage to be treated beyond the point where their care would represent a loss, rather than a profit, for the institution. It is well known that intensive care units are hospitals' biggest money-spinners. This explains their proliferation during the expansionist 1960s and 1970s. But where MediCal patients, for example, are not generating but instead are losing income for the hospital, it would be advantageous to the institution to get them out of the ICU as quickly as possible. This could lead to morally as well as medically inappropriate decisions about the limitation of therapy.

Of these two possible scenarios—the hospital's desire to avoid bad publicity and its incentive to reduce ICU costs—the former is the more likely to occur. Defensively concerned to avoid malpractice litigation, hospitals have disregarded patient autonomy, expressed either directly or through surrogates, by refusing to allow the withholding or withdrawal of life-sustaining therapies in at least three cases. They are the New Jersey Supreme Court cases of Kathleen Farrell, a 37-year-old competent patient terminally ill with amyotrophic lateral sclerosis (ALS); Hilda Peter, a 65-year-old incompetent, institutionalized patient with a legally valid directive to physicians stating her wishes in advance about limiting medical care; and Nancy Ellen Jobes, an incompetent institutionalized patient who had no credible advance directive.

In each case, the court upheld the best interests of the patient against those of the institution, giving weight to patient autonomy or the presumed autonomous wishes of the patient concerned. But isolated court decisions, not binding in other jurisdictions, are inadequate to deal with institutionalized intrusion into the decision-making process. Only resolute legislative action can nullify this economic incentive and establish the principle of autonomy in its morally appropriate place. Until that happens, sounder advice for physicians and for patients or their surrogates can usually be obtained from disinterested legal counsel than from the hospital's own lawyers. Inevitably, hospital lawyers tend to be conservative.

Society

The last column in Table 9-1 represents society. Society impinges in many ways upon those involved in decisions to limit therapy in the intensive care unit. Its primary impact is felt in terms of economic and legal constraints. From an economic perspective, society's interest in limiting therapy is grounded in the principle of distributive justice: the need to allocate fairly among the many claimants for them the limited intensive care resources available.

If economic considerations are to enter into decisions made about intensive care, as inevitably they must, they need to take effect at the policy level, beforehand, rather than in the clinical situation, after the fact. This applies to both institutional and societal budgetary reductions. Inevitably, this will lead to the increased bureaucratization of the practice of medicine. The concomitant danger is that policies applicable across the board will not prove flexible enough to meet the unique needs of individuals. Only those with strong convictions about the respect due to patients will be able to temper justice with mercy, and thus make "the system" function in more, rather than in less, humane fashion.

Court decisions and legislation will also have an increasing impact on decisions to limit therapy in the intensive care unit. Let us hope that the guiding principle will continue to be that of patient autonomy and that physicians acting out of respect for patient autonomy will be exonerated from all later legal repercussions. If this assurance is not given, self-interest on the part of caregivers is bound to outweigh concerns about upholding the right of individual patients to be self-determining, so far as possible, in matters relating to their medical care.

Further court precedents are inevitable. One recently handed down is the verdict in the case of Elizabeth Bouvia, the cerebral palsy victim who in 1983 unsuccessfully sought court permission to starve herself to death at Riverside, California, General Hospital–University Medical Center. Subsequently, she was again admitted to a southern California hospital. Once more, the physicians treating her refused her request for removal of a life-sustaining feeding tube. Yet again, she petitioned the court to order it removed.

Her motive in now wanting the feeding tube removed, she claimed, was not to starve herself to death: it was merely to be able to choose her own treatment. She felt that her caloric intake was sufficient to sustain her life without intravenous hydration or nasogastric tube nutrition. Her physicians disagreed. Her "continued refusal to eat adequate food was viewed by the staff as an attempt at suicide starvation," county attorneys for the hospital stated in their court papers. This time, the court ruled in Ms. Bouvia's favor, and the nasogastric feeding tube was withdrawn. Subsequently, when her physicians sought to deny her intravenous morphine for control of her constant pain, Ms. Bouvia again petitioned the court. The court upheld her claim. She now receives food by mouth and morphine intravenously, and appears not to be in imminent danger of dying.

As we shall see in Chapter 12, it is possible to identify five factors that continually create fresh ethical quandaries in the contemporary practice of medicine: the discovery of new diseases; the advent of new technologies; novel legal judgments and legislative measures; emerging economic constraints; and sociological phenomena, such as nurses developing and asserting their own distinctive professional identity. All five factors conjoin in the modern intensive care unit, so that it is here that the ethical issues are presented most acutely and with the utmost poignancy. It is possible, however, to approach these problems in a principled way. It is also possible to identify those who, potentially, are able to participate in decisions to limit therapy, and to suggest what their respective contributions ought to be, and why.

Let us return to the case that introduced this chapter.

Jerry's autonomy was upheld—by his wife and children, his nursing and medical caregivers, myself as ethics consultant, the hospital administration representative, and the hospital's legal counsel. Defensively compelling him to remain on a ventilator would not have cured his disease; it would only have violated his sense of self and the values by which he had lived for 48 *years. Beneficence does not require physicians to attempt the impossible. Nonmaleficence does allow for the introduction of compassion and choice into an otherwise sterile and highly technological environment. And justice would not have been served by expending close to $2,000 a day on intensive care to prolong the process of Jerry's inevitable demise.*

In the evening, two days after his decision, Jerry asked that he be given time with his wife and children to say his goodbyes before being sedated. He requested that when he was asleep he be withdrawn from the breathing machine. Should he experience any discomfort as he died of oxygen starvation, he wanted it to be controlled with medication.

His wishes were honored, down to the last detail. Four hours after being removed from the ventilator, Jerry died. His was a painless, and apparently peaceful, death. His wife was with him throughout the hours of his dying, as were his nurses and those who had provided him with medical care and emotional, spiritual, and ethical support while he was alive. His story bears testimony to the fact that death can occur humanely and with dignity, even within an intensive care unit in a major medical center.

10

Assisted Suicide[1]

"**W**hen my first wife could no longer bear the pain and deterioration of her body and the distressed quality of her life from cancer, she asked me to help her end her life. It was both a logical and a poignant request. . . .

"I remembered a young doctor whom I had met many years before while reporting on medical matters for my newspaper. Over several months he had supplied me with vital—and secret—information on a political matter which affected the health professions. Partly due to my articles in the Sunday Times (London), written extensively as a result of this doctor's briefings, there were salutary reforms in the health service that benefited patients.

"So I called 'Joe' and asked if we could meet. He invited me to his consulting rooms, for he had by now become an eminent physician with a lucrative practice. As prestigious and powerful as he was, he still had not lost the compassion and humanity that I had noted in earlier years. I told him how seriously ill Jean was and of her desire to die soon. He questioned me closely on the state of the disease, its effects on her, and what treatments she had undergone.

"Once he heard that some of her bones were breaking at the slightest sudden movement, he stopped the conversation. 'There's no quality of life left for her,' he said, getting up from his desk and striding to his medicine cabinet. He studied the contents for a minute.

"I don't want to give you something that has by law to be entered in the poisons register,' he said. 'I'll make a call.' Joe then telephoned the chief pharmacist at the hospital to which he was attached. 'The wife of a friend of *mine wants to end her life because of advanced cancer,' he said. 'What do you recommend to use?'*

"There followed a conversation that was too technical for me to understand. When it ended, Joe returned to his drug cabinet, did some mixing of pills, and handed a vial to me, explaining that the capsules should be emptied into a sweet drink to reduce the bitter taste.

"'This is strictly between you and me,' he said, looking straight into my eyes.

"'You have my word that no one will ever know of your part in this,' I promised. I thanked him and left.

"A few weeks later, when Jean knew that the time had come, she asked me for the drugs. As wrenching as it was, I had to agree. We spent the morning reminiscing about our twenty-one years together. Then, dissolving the pills in some coffee, we said our last goodbyes. I watched as Jean picked up the coffee and drank it down. She barely had time to murmur, 'Goodbye, my love,' before falling asleep. Fifty minutes later she stopped breathing."[2]

In Chapter 9, there was a deliberate omission of an important ethical issue occasionally confronted by those providing medical and family care to people who are terminally ill: that of assisting them to commit suicide. This topic is the subject of proposed initiatives in the states of Florida and California to legalize the enabling of those who are terminally ill to end their own lives and is of wide interest. Although my primary intent is to provide an ethical perspective on helping terminally ill persons who want to die, let us begin the analysis by reflecting briefly on suicide in general.

With respect to suicide, two moral principles are typically in opposition to one another. On the one hand, there is the principle of *autonomy*[3] which requires that, consistent with the welfare of others and so far as possible, persons ought to be respected and treated as self-determining moral agents. A caregiver focusing exclusively on the principle of autonomy could conclude that the wish of a woman to choose death rather than life ought to be respected, so long as there was evidence to suggest that she was indeed mentally competent. In the case of the fully rational person, suicide may logically be regarded as the ultimate expression of autonomy. Such an individual manifests the will to be self-determining, not only in matters of life, but also in the manner and timing of death. Socrates is in this sense the prototypical autonomous man.

On the other hand, there is also the principle of *beneficence* to be reckoned with. Beneficence imposes on us a duty to benefit others when in a position to do so, and readily invites paternalistic behavior. In the ethical literature, paternalism refers

> to practices that restrict the liberty of individuals without their consent, where the justification for such actions is either the prevention of some harm they will do themselves or the production of some benefit for them they would not otherwise secure.[4]

In the normal course of events, it would be instinctive for the physician to act paternalistically and beneficently by attempting to save the life of someone wanting to kill himself. Observance of the duty of beneficence would compel a physician to assume that a suicidal individual was not rational, and to act paternalistically to prevent him from harming himself. This, in turn, reflects a value judgment: no one in his right mind would want to kill himself; to want to kill oneself, one must be mentally off-balance or emotionally unhinged—at least temporarily.

That this value judgment is widely shared within our society prompts the conclusion, for example, that whenever someone is brought into an emergency room as the result of an overdose of medication, such a person was mentally incompetent at the time the overdose was taken. The principle of beneficence, paternalistically applied, as is inevitable in an emergency situation, requires cardio-pulmonary resuscitation, the stomach being pumped out, the drug ingested being identified, and immediate steps being taken to counter its effects; these include, if necessary, intubation, ventilatory support, renal dialysis, and other intensive care interventions.

In the context of suicide in general, the principles of autonomy and beneficence are antithetical. The wish to respect others as self-determining moral agents, as long as their actions are not infringing upon the liberty of others or causing others harm and as long as they are mentally competent and rational, is inherently opposed to the duty to benefit them by preventing them from being harmed. These two principles cannot be applied simultaneously and without conflict, any more than the imperatives to preserve life and alleviate suffering can be invoked concurrently in the final stages of a terminal illness. The question, then, is how to rank autonomy and beneficence in dealing with the suicidal individual, and on what basis.

In response to this question, I shall propose and then develop two theses. The first is that in the absence of an underlying terminal and painful disease process, the principle of beneficence ought *prima facie* to take precedence over the principle of autonomy in responding to suicidal attempts or desires. And the second is that when the suicidal person does have an underlying terminal and painful medical condition, or is in an advanced state of decrepitude, and is mentally competent and fully rational, the principle of autonomy ought *prima facie* to assume priority over that of beneficence.

Suicide in the Absence of a Terminal Illness

The foundation on which the first thesis rests is a cultural value judgment that in the absence of some major misfortune, medical or otherwise, and on balance, life is preferable to death. Obviously, this value judgment is not endorsed by everyone. Suicides occur frequently. And it is disturbing, to say the least, that data beginning to be accumulated indicate the growing estrangement of significant numbers of young people from this shared value.[5] As an example, here are two verses from a poem written by a seventeen-year-old boy from an affluent home a year ago:

> Inside my head is pounding
> Been hurting me for weeks
> I've got to find salvation
> I've got to find some peace.
>
> I just now realized
> I have new decisions to make:
> What building shall I jump from
> What pills should I take?

Despite being scholarly, athletic, musically gifted, handsome, and in other ways remarkably talented, a year after writing these lines Todd leaped to his death from a high-rise building on the campus where he was a student. He was one of approximately six thousand who succeeded in killing themselves out of the estimated four hundred thousand young people who attempt suicide each year.[6] A recent spate of group teen-age suicides and attempted suicides is indicative of how profoundly alienated many young people are from the dominant values of our culture.

The values and value judgments which, as we have seen, enter decisively into the ethical decisions we make, whether consciously or unconsciously, are correlated closely with deeply held metaphysical beliefs. Those who stand within the Judeo-Christian tradition and affirm life with all its problems and difficulties to be an essentially good gift from the hand of God will want to value life above death, even in the worst of times. Whether or not they actually succeed in doing this is another matter. Those who, although less directly connected to any religious tradition, are nevertheless able to affirm an evolutionary and optimistic world view—the American dream—will also be inclined, on the whole and except under extreme stress, to value life above death, adversity notwithstanding.

In both instances, value judgments are being made. Obviously, at times and in both groups there will be exceptions, those unable to continue to uphold these values who choose death above life. The young, growing up in the shadow of nuclear proliferation and potential annihilation, are less easily able to believe that good will automatically triumph over evil; that, inevitably, light will drive back darkness. With the beliefs and value systems of previous generations no longer accessible to them, it should not surprise us that a disturbingly large number of young people do not instinctively value life above death even in the absence of poignant personal affliction.

The dominant value system in our society, however, affirms life, not death. When someone is threatening, or attempting, to commit suicide, beneficence would immediately assume priority over autonomy, so long as there were no known underlying terminal disease process, increasing physical or mental decrepitude, or unmitigable pain. Our value system would cause us to presume that the suicidal person's competency had been compromised and that the wish or action to end his or her own life was not truly autonomous. The intention of intervening would be not only to prevent the wish from being translated into the deed, but also to provide him with such appropriate therapy, counseling, or support as would serve eventually to remove the impediments to competency. To restore the patient to substantial autonomy could lead to a reaffirmation of the goodness of life.

A related assumption in ranking beneficence over autonomy is that if both interventions, the medical and the psychiatric, were effective, the suicidal person would later provide future consent to what had been done to frustrate his death wish and restore him to competency.

Once the crisis is past, it is anticipated that the formerly suicidal person will be glad and grateful that someone intervened paternalistically and beneficently to avert death and to renew his perspective. That there is often empirical evidence, *ex post facto*, indicating that such an assumption was in fact correct further strengthens the bias in favor of subordinating autonomy to beneficence.[7]

Suicide in a Situation of Terminal Illness

There is, however, a growing societal recognition of a category of people who constitute a valid exception to the usual evaluation of and response to suicide. When someone is afflicted with an underlying terminal condition, is in a state of advanced physical or mental decrepitude, and/or is in unmitigable pain, the distinction drawn in Chapter 9 commands attention: There is a difference between being able to extend life with all that makes life full and good and merely prolonging an inevitable and painful process of dying. If this distinction is legitimate, there may well be a point beyond which life is no longer to be valued above death. Now the principle of autonomy may in good conscience be ranked above the principle of beneficence, so long as the person wishing to end his or her life is at the time mentally competent and rational, and so long as all possible steps have been taken to minimize the ensuing harm to others.[8]

This chain of reasoning undergirds the second thesis. Providing that someone who is talking about ending her own life

- is either terminally ill or irreversibly sinking into physical or mental decrepitude

- is in unmitigable pain—whether physical or psychological, or both

- is clearly rational and competent

- and has attempted to mitigate the harmful effects of her action on those who will survive her by seeking to alleviate the guilt they will predictably experience,

then it is morally acceptable to rank the principle of autonomy above the principle of beneficence. This means that the paternalistic impulse to intervene in order to prevent the suicide will need to be restrained, and that the suicidal intent may now be regarded as the final expression of autonomy and respected as such.

A caveat is in order here: theologically speaking, suicide may be regarded as a predictable response to the breakdown or absence of faith, of being able to affirm the essential meaningfulness of human existence, especially in the face of pain; hope, in terms of being able to look to the future with confidence and with courage, despite all present distress; and love, being able to affirm the self as inherently lovable and worthy and on this basis being able to receive from and proffer others a similar affirmation.

When the experience of terminal illness and the pain sometimes associated with it have ceased to be meaningful; when the future is perceived as holding nothing but further affliction and debilitation, and there no longer appear to be grounds for confidence and courage with respect to what is yet to be; and when it not only becomes impossible to affirm the present self as worthy but also seems that significant others no longer care or are interested in whether or not the terminally ill person cares about them, then the wish to choose death above life is altogether reasonable and predictable.[9]

Before simply giving permission to someone who is terminally ill and in intractable pain to take the fateful step of translating the suicidal impulse into action, it is first of all necessary, from a theological perspective, for the caregiver to attempt to help the terminally ill and suicidal person to find or regain a sense of the meaningfulness of all human experience, suffering included. It is to endeavor to facilitate in her the capacity to look to the future with confidence and with courage, extending her vision, if need be, beyond the horizons of time to the limitless vista of eternity. And it is to try to instill in her the conviction that she is essentially lovable, no matter how dramatically her outward appearance may be deteriorating from one day to the next.

Such an effort may or may not require the use of religious representatives or language. Spirituality is a category of human experience broader and more universal than religion, yet inclusive of it. It is possible to speak of faith, hope, and love in either religious or secular metaphors. Which are employed will depend on the belief and value system of the suicidal person.

Only after seriously striving to enable the dying person to find or regain faith, hope, and love, and not succeeding is it morally allowable to acquiesce in his wish to choose death rather than life. Only then is it ethically permissible to restrain oneself from the beneficent and paternalistic impulse to frustrate his death wish. And only then is it ethically appropriate to allow autonomy to be the more important principle.

It is one thing to acquiesce; it is another to assist. Assenting to a terminally ill person's desire to end his life may be morally appropriate, especially where the conditions outlined above have been satisfied. Can the same be said of assisting? The first question to be addressed is this: Is there a moral difference between saying to someone who wishes to commit suicide "I'll not stop you" and "I'll help you"? I believe there is. In saying "I'll not stop you," I may be expressing respect for a state of mind, a belief system, or an intention to act in a certain way that I myself do not endorse, yet which, for the person concerned and in the circumstances described, may seem to be appropriate. For me to go on to say "I'll help you" would require a much higher level of personal endorsement of the other's state of mind, belief system, or intention to act.

There is a difference between respect and assent. I respect the views of Creationists, Marxists, and Jehovah's Witnesses. I do not assent to them. I may or may not assent to the suicidal desire being expressed although I may respect it. If I am unable to assent to the suicidal fixation, even though I may respect it, there is absolutely no moral obligation upon me to go beyond saying "I'll not stop you" to "I'll help you." To be compelled to do so would compromise my own autonomy, my own belief and value systems, my own understanding of the meaning of faith, hope, and love. The principle of beneficence does not impose on me a duty to act in a way that the patient may regard as beneficial but which I myself believe to be harmful.

It seems to me that a crucial point emerges from this distinction. If one were to go beyond saying "I'll not stop you" to promise "I'll help you" one would be acting autonomously rather than because of any perceived extrinsic moral obligation or duty. The principle of beneficence does not extend this far, especially within the context of the practice of medicine. Were one to help someone to die, it could only be because of an intrinsic sense of compassion.

There is no extrinsic moral obligation or duty compelling one person to help another to accomplish his own death, and, conversely, the person contemplating suicide has no concomitant right to help. Only duties correspond to rights; only rights entail duties. The Internal Revenue Service has the right to exact a levy on one's income; paying income tax is one's concomitant duty. In returning to the California public school system one's state income tax rebate, one acts voluntarily, expressing one's autonomy in so doing, and not because of a legal duty extrinsically imposed.

Hence, assisting someone who is terminally ill and in intractable pain to end her life may be something a caregiver will choose to do out of generosity, compassion, or a sense of common humanity. If the caregiver were to afford help, it would be because he or she not only respected but also endorsed the suicidal intention. It would not be because the patient has some right to such assistance which, in turn, the caregiver has a duty to render.

The factors which may lead one to assent to views which one may already respect are many and various: the quality of one's relationship with the person now wishing to end his life; the degree to which one shares his values, beliefs, and reasoned convictions about the preference for death over life in the circumstances he is presently experiencing; the inability of the person wanting to die to accomplish his own death without assistance; and one's capacity to provide the assistance being asked for.

Where the relationship between the potential helper and the terminally ill patient is extremely close; where there is a high degree of assent to the patient's values, beliefs, and convictions; where he or she cannot die without assistance; and where the potential helper is, in fact, in a position to provide the kind of assistance being sought, then, while there may be no duty to assist, it would be difficult to sustain the argument that it would be immoral freely to choose to help and to bear the consequences.

Bioethicist Tristram Englehardt, both a physician and a philosopher, ventures even further. He argues in support of the right of individuals to commit suicide, and then concludes:

> Insofar as individuals possess this right for themselves, they should have as well the right to be aided by others.[10]

This does not necessarily follow. The logic is faulty. It is not enough simply to draw from the argument that persons have a "right" to die the conclusion that therefore, automatically, they "have as well the right to be aided by others." I prefer not to use the word "rights" in this context, for rights imply corresponding duties. Where does this right come from? What is its source? The absence of answers to these questions makes it impossible to assert with any confidence that there is a duty to provide such aid. Nevertheless, as has been suggested, a caregiver may voluntarily choose to provide assistance as a freely offered act of kindness—a very different matter.

The motivation of the potential helper is, of course, crucial. Where the motive is disinterested kindness, compassion, or humaneness, it may be morally acceptable to help someone wishing to die to achieve a painless death. But were the motive one of wanting to inherit or in other ways to benefit personally, this would obviously cast an altogether different light on the assistance being given. Usually, motivation cannot be properly assessed until after the fact, which is what juries and judges attempt to do. Helping another person to die should therefore, never be given legal sanction. Accordingly, there may be legal and other consequences to be borne by anyone helping another to die.

Kinds of Assistance

This brings us to a final issue: the nature of the assistance that might be given were one to be morally convinced of the appropriateness of helping someone who wanted to commit suicide but was unable to accomplish this for himself. Various types of assistance may be imagined, ranging from the seemingly innocuous to those far more serious and fraught with risk. The options would include:

(a) *Encouragement.* Removing obstacles in the way of the person wishing to end his or her life; for example, by reassuring him that he will not be judged and damned by God for so acting, or by suggesting that if the roles were reversed, one would oneself possibly be contemplating suicide

(b) *Information* of the sort provided by the Hemlock Society or Exit about how to accomplish one's own death in the least traumatic and most effective manner[11]

(c) *Provision or procurement of the necessary means* if the suicidal person is and would otherwise be without the means to end his life—a physician, for example, writing for the patient a prescription for pain medication, an overdose of which could cause his death

(d) *Helping to administer the means to be employed:* mixing the lethal dose and raising it to the lips of the person wishing to die, or holding the gun to the suicidal person's head and placing his finger on the trigger

(e) *Actually killing* the person wishing to die, at his request— for example, by smothering, shooting, or poisoning. The line between assisted suicide of this type and mercy killing at the request of the person wishing to die is blurred. I find it almost impossible to draw a moral distinction between them.

This spectrum of possible forms of help ranges from category (a), requiring relatively slight involvement on the part of the helper and little more than empathy and a nonjudgmental attitude, to category (e), where the involvement of the helper would be major and would require him or her actually to take the life of another human being. Moral arguments could be made in support of each option. How far along the spectrum from (a) toward (e) the helper will be willing to go will depend on the factors previously mentioned.

What is obvious is that the consequences of helping become much more serious as one moves from (a) through (e). Providing the sorts of assistance suggested in (d) and (e) could result in the helper having to face criminal or civil charges. However, the helper who deeply loves the person wishing to die, shares his beliefs and values, is persuaded by his reasons for wanting to end it all, and is in a position to help, both emotionally and practically, may be willing to risk such serious consequences and to go as far as (d) or (e), where the friend or relative wishing to die is entirely incapable of accomplishing his own death. Were she so to act, this would be an act of courage and compassion of the highest order.

Legal Implications

Some conclusions of a legal nature follow from the argument that has been made, and a few recommendations suggest themselves. A range of possible responses open to people who, for whatever reason, no longer regard life as a benefit and choose, rationally and competently, to act autonomously and commit suicide follows.

In the case of those not afflicted with an underlying terminal illness, nor in a state of advanced decrepitude, the presumption is that their competency is in some way compromised or impaired and that, therefore, the principle of beneficence, paternalistically applied, ought to take precedence over the principle of autonomy. If it is later established that with full rationality and competency, death was still being valued above life, and every possible effort had been made to enable the suicidal person to view life as a benefit rather than as a detriment, then reluctantly one would have to acquiesce in his or her decision to die—on the basis of the principle of autonomy. It follows that if such a suicidal attempt were unsuccessful, the person concerned should not be subject to criminal charges.

In the case of the terminally ill or those in an advanced and irreversible state of decrepitude who are suffering unbearably yet are rational and competent, the customary ranking of principles ought to be reversed, with autonomy now taking priority over beneficence. This is why I object to criminal charges being brought against those who unsuccessfully attempt to end their own lives in circumstances of terminal illness or advanced decrepitude and unmitigable pain, after every effort has been made to minimize for the survivors the untoward consequences of the act.

An even more difficult question is what legal penalties, if any, ought to be borne by those who assist people to end their lives. In my view, those who encourage or provide information to those wishing to die ought not to be subject to prosecution; helping someone to accomplish his own death or actually killing him at his request ought to be subject to legal penalties of a special kind. And procuring for someone wishing to die the means necessary to do this falls into an ambiguous category for the following reasons: encouraging or providing information to someone wishing to die, in the circumstances we have considered, represents a modest step from acquiescence to assent. Both forms of assistance enhance the autonomy of the terminally ill person who feels unable any longer to continue the struggle to survive. It would be hypocritical to argue that while autonomy ought to be respected, acts which enhance autonomy ought to be subject to criminal charges.

Directly assisting someone to die, however, or actually killing him at his own request is a far more serious action and susceptible to more serious kinds of abuse by those, for example, whose motivation is not altruistic and disinterested but self-serving. Because it is usually possible to be certain about motivation only when an after-the-fact assessment has been made, such actions ought always to be subject to legal scrutiny. This would require criminal charges being brought against those so assisting or killing. However, in those cases where the motivation was seen to be manifestly altruistic and disinterested, the penalties ought to be nominal or nonexistent. To subject persons found guilty of killing for reasons of compassion to the same penalties as those found guilty of first- or second-degree murder seems excessive, unjust, and unnecessary.

This leaves the ambiguous category of those who procure for someone wishing to end her own life in the circumstances we are describing the means she is unable to obtain for herself. Here it appears that the criminality, if any, of the assistance given should depend on a case-by-case assessment of what help was actually afforded. A physician who appropriately prescribes sleeping pills for a terminally ill patient ought not to be subject to criminal charges if the patient swallows all the pills at once in order to commit suicide. On the other hand, a physician who inappropriately prescribes medications the sole effect of which would be to cause death ought to be subject to criminal investigation. Again, if it should subsequently be established that the motivation was transparently compassionate, the penalties should be nominal or nonexistent. Unless legal penalties are possible, even in cases where it was appropriate to help someone to die, the door could easily be opened to the inappropriate shortening of others' lives.

This leads to some final recommendations. Laws treating suicide as a criminal offense ought to be eliminated. Laws forbidding the provision of assistance to those terminally ill yet competent wishing to die ought to be struck down where the assistance is merely that of offering encouragement or providing information. And laws forbidding the provision of other kinds of assistance to persons wishing to die, as in (c), (d), and (e) above, ought to remain in place. However, the penalties ought to be reduced to the point where they are nominal or nonexistent in those cases where it is clearly established that the motivation of the helper was not at all sinister, but unambiguously reflected compassion and love.[12]

Derek Humphry's first wife, Jean, died "as she wished and as she deserved." Dr. Joe broke the law by prescribing the drugs that ended her life. Humphry committed the crime of assisting a suicide. No wonder he asks the following three questions, pertinent now as they were several years ago, here as well as where the incident occurred:

"Did Dr. Joe and I commit truly felonious, culpable crimes and did we deserve punishment?

"Aren't these archaic laws ready to be changed to ways befitting modern understanding and morality?

"Not everyone has as good a friend in the medical profession as I had. Why should caring doctors like Dr. Joe have to take such appalling risks?"

How our society will respond to Humphry's questions is less important than the resolve to address them. And since the topic of assisted suicide is of such crucial importance, whatever answers we formulate must display reasoned consideration and be publicly defensible, rather than reflect emotion alone.

11

The AIDS Crisis

Dr. Lois Dorsey, a psychiatry resident, was paged by an intern from the Medical Intensive Care Unit (MICU) for an emergency psychiatry consultation. Gary Davidson, a twenty-eight-year-old gay man, had been hospitalized eleven days before for a first episode of Pneumocystis carinii pneumonia (PCP). One week earlier he had been told that the presumptive diagnosis for his illness was Acquired Immunodeficiency Syndrome (AIDS).

On the day Dr. Dorsey was called, the medical team discussed with Mr. Davidson the need for a Swann-Ganz catheter, which would be inserted in his pulmonary artery. Mr. Davidson refused permission for placement of the catheter and requested that medical treatment be stopped. "Take the tubes away and let me die with dignity," he declared.

The medical team discussed in detail with Mr. Davidson, his lover, and his parents and sister his clinical status and prognosis: Mr. Davidson had, they believed, a 50 percent chance of surviving the current illness. However, people with AIDS rarely survive more than two years, and Mr. Davidson could expect several bouts of severe illness during his remaining lifespan. They also pointed out that rapid advances were being made in understanding the pathophysiology of AIDS and offered the possibility of future treatment as a result of current research efforts.

With the support of his lover and family, Mr. Davidson continued to insist on cessation of treatment, citing as his reasons "quality of life" and "the right to die with dignity." In the presence of witnesses he signed a living will and statement of competency. The legal formalities were carried out; however, for "legal reasons" and "completeness," before complying with the patient's request, the medical team was waiting for a psychiatric assessment.

Dr. Dorsey reviewed Mr. Davidson's records and interviewed him. Mr. Davidson reaffirmed his belief that quality of life was more important than *quantity of life and that he wished to die with dignity. He admitted that he was feeling pain, fear, loss of control, extreme discomfort on the respirator, and sleepiness. He added that he was distressed by his inability to eat while on the respirator. When Dr. Dorsey asked how he might feel should he recover from the pneumonia, the patient noted that he knew he had AIDS and that he would die within one or two years. Therefore, he said, he did not deserve to take up a bed in the hospital and continue to receive medical treatment that could better benefit another patient.*

The patient had no psychiatric history and had never attempted suicide. He had never had any personal experience with death or dying among family or friends. He could not speak because of the respirator tubes, but he communicated by writing notes and nodding his head. He was alert, not disoriented; wrote clearly and logically; and initiated his own statements and topics for the interview. He was not tearful but appeared anxious. In his own eyes he did not want to commit suicide but wanted to be allowed to die.

Dr. Dorsey concluded that the patient showed no evidence of confusion, psychosis, or delusional thinking, but that he did show symptoms consistent with depression, probably secondary to his underlying medical condition.

Mr. Davidson, then, was legally competent, understood the consequences of his decision to refuse treatment, and had the support of those closest to him. Yet, because of his age and depression, the availability of treatment for his current illness, and the possibility that some treatment for AIDS may become available within the next few years, Dr. Dorsey hesitated. Should Mr. Davidson's treatment be stopped as he wished?[1]

The familiar ethical dilemma of autonomy versus beneficence surfaces again in this particular case. But there are other issues generated by the AIDS epidemic that must be addressed: among these are professional responsibilities to AIDS patients;[2] public health and civil liberties;[3] the socioeconomic impact of AIDS;[4] and the risk to insurers.[5] This is not an exhaustive list of the ethical quandaries which this new disease has generated. It is possible to deal with only a selected few within the space of a single chapter, and what follows is more in the way of an introductory overview than a definitive treatment. But first, some historical and demographic details are necessary to put the epidemic into perspective.

Since it was first recognized in July of 1981 as a new and fatal disease, AIDS has spread at an alarming rate through the male homosexual and intravenous-drug-using populations. Its transmission, by blood transfusions and via bisexual men, into the heterosexual populations has been less dramatic, but nonetheless allows no room for complacency. Corresponding to the geographic distribution of the high-risk populations, AIDS has been most prevalent on the East and West coasts—particularly in the New York and San Francisco regions. This is expected to change in the next five years. While AIDS will continue to present an enormous health care problem on both coasts, it is outside the New York and San Francisco areas that the highest growth rates are anticipated. This is evident from the latest Centers for Disease Control projections.

Table 11-1: Centers for Disease Control Projections of AIDS Prevalence*

Location	1986	1991	1991 (low)	1991 (high)
New York	7,553	20,532	13,594	24,638
San Francisco	3,014	13,920	9,216	16,704
Other U.S.	20,513	139,548	92,390	167,458
Total U.S.	31,080	174,000	115,200	208,800

*Source: W. M. Morgan, AIDS program, Center for Infectious Diseases Centers for Disease Control.

There is some evidence to suggest that the rate at which AIDS is spreading is slowing down, largely as a result of educational endeavors and resulting behavioral changes. Nevertheless, the prospects are still alarming. By 1991 the medical care costs for persons with AIDS are likely to exceed the medical care costs both for patients with cancer of the digestive system, of the lungs, and of the breast and for those with end-stage renal disease. Only injuries sustained in automobile accidents will command more of our medical care resources than AIDS![6] For the foreseeable future, AIDS will remain close to the top of the list of medical care problems in the United States. What devastation it will be causing in Africa and Asia can only be dimly imagined. It is against this background that we go on to look at five selected ethical issues generated by this dread disease.

Responsibilities of Health Care Providers to AIDS Patients

In November, 1987, the *New York Times* reported the following statement by the American Medical Association:

The American Medical Association declared today [November 12, 1987] that doctors had an ethical obligation to care for people with AIDS as well as for those who had been infected with the virus but showed no symptoms.

The statement was the first pronouncement by the organization on the duties of doctors in the AIDS epidemic. It came amid reports that a small number of doctors had refused to treat patients with acquired immunodeficiency syndrome, a disease for which there is no cure.

The association, the voice of organized medicine in the United States, said "A physician may not ethically refuse to treat a patient whose condition is within the physician's current realm of competence solely because the patient has been infected with the AIDS virus."[7]

This statement was issued after more than six years of ambivalence and silence, during which time twelve health care workers, worldwide, had become infected with the AIDS virus. It does not address the moral issue of physicians neither refusing to treat nor actually treating, exemplified by attending physicians simply delegating to medical residents the direct care of patients with AIDS. Neither, of course, does it speak to the professional responsibilities of others—notably registered nurses—more immediately involved than physicians in caring for AIDS patients.

Until the end of 1986, the AMA was silent on the subject of physicians' professional obligations to patients with AIDS. Then, on December 1, 1986, the AMA made a brief pronouncement in which the medical profession's long-standing tradition of caring for contagious patients was acknowledged but which went on to allow that "not everyone is emotionally able to care for patients with AIDS."[8] This, taken in conjunction with Section VI of the AMA's Principles of Medical Ethics, continued to provide physicians with a highly ambiguous moral mandate. This section reads: "A physician shall, in the provision of appropriate patient care, except in emergencies, be free to choose whom to serve."[9]

In the meantime, many physicians, dentists, nurses, dieticians, and technicians were refusing to deal with AIDS patients. Sometimes, the refusal was explicit; at other times, it was implicit in the way attending physicians, for example, would themselves avoid all direct contact with AIDS simply by delegating the care of infected patients to the medical house staff over whom they exercised authority. For the most part, this was prompted by fear. For the same reason, some mortuaries were refusing to provide services to the victims of AIDS. Partly to protect themselves, but perhaps also in order to humiliate and intimidate those with whom they had little empathy, several police departments were at the same time issuing yellow rubber gloves to be worn by officers charged with crowd control during gay rights demonstrations!

Virtually all confirmed infections of health care workers occurred after an accidental injury, most often from a needle that had been used on a patient. But fear of infection is not the only motive for the refusal of some caregivers to be involved with AIDS patients. In the case of many physicians and nurses, the phenomenon of "AIDS burnout,"[10] resulting "from too many intense, emotion-filled relationships with young, dying patients,"[11] is a compelling reason for withdrawing from the front lines in the fight against AIDS. In the case of others, homophobia (prejudice against and fear of homosexuals) is probably at the root of their unwillingness to become involved. The problem of "the hateful patient" is not unique to AIDS patients who are either homosexuals or intravenous drug addicts and obvious targets for prejudice; it manifests itself also in the treatment (or non-treatment) of alcoholics, the grossly obese, the non-compliant patient, and felons.

What, then, *is* the moral responsibility of caregivers toward AIDS patients? It is impossible to answer this question in the abstract or in general terms. Each professional has to decide for her- or himself what the answer shall be. However, a personal opinion and the reasons behind it may be helpful.

My own view is based on the notion of professional responsibility. The physician as member of the medical profession is not the same as the physician as entrepreneur or the physician as technician. As the root of the word "professional" attests, members of "the three learned professions"—originally divinity, law, and medicine—professed something: they professed certain skills, and they professed to practice them with disinterested motivation and with concern, not primarily for their own benefit, but for the benefit of others.

So long as the physician or the nurse is committed to medicine or to nursing as a profession with a sense of vocation and not as a business venture or as a technical endeavor, then a primary concern to benefit others is expected as a corollary. This would require impartial treatment even of "the hateful patient," as it would the acceptance of risk. The willingness to place the well-being of others above their own safety or private biases is the price members of the health care professions pay for the honor and respect accorded them by the wider society.

Normatively speaking, this view is grounded in an ethics of virtue.[12] It applies not only to physicians but to other professionals such as nurses, social workers, and chaplains as well. Steven Miles and Abigail Zuger, who have consistently addressed the issue of professional responsibility to AIDS patients, make the ethics-of-virtue argument in these terms:

> A virtue-based medical ethic has powerful implications for the care of contagious patients in general, and HIV-infected patients in particular. It recognizes that all HIV-infected persons are in need of the healing art—for counseling and reassurance, if nothing else. It mandates, as well, that because of their prior voluntary commitment to the *professio* of healing, physicians are obliged to undertake the *officia* of caring for these patients. Individual physicians who decline to perform these *officia* are falling short of an excellence in practice implicit in their professional commitment.[13]

However, even a virtuous professional can legitimately claim to have reached a point of such emotional and spiritual depletion as to make it difficult to the point of impossibility to continue in the front lines. Burnout can and does occur—even to the most dedicated of caregivers. Once the point of burnout has been reached, it becomes morally appropriate for the professional to place her or his own well-being above that of others, if only temporarily, for the sake of being able to continue the fight another day. This is simple prudence. It is an honorable motive for leaving the battle to others, and is perhaps the only motive for so doing that can be morally justified.

Public Health and Civil Liberties

Given the facts that it is possible to test only for exposure to the AIDS virus and not for the disease itself; that the simpler and cheaper test for exposure to the human immunodeficiency virus (HIV) yields approximately 5 percent false positives; and that the incubation period for the virus may be anything between two and six months, making possible several false negatives, ought testing to be mandatory or merely voluntary? Should there be mandatory reporting of those who test HIV-positive? And should the behavior of those who have tested positive for the virus somehow be circumscribed, for example, by means of tattooing, computerized registration, or quarantining? These are but three of the many ethical issues raised by the AIDS epidemic which reflect an indissoluble tension between individual liberties and the common good. Each of them warrants a brief exploration.

Testing for HIV Infection

There are two tests currently available to ascertain whether or not an individual has been exposed to the human immunodeficiency virus. The simpler and cheaper test, the Elisa, can, in up to one out of every twenty cases, falsely indicate that the person tested has been exposed to the AIDS virus. These are the so-called "false positives." If a second, more expensive test, the Western blot, is done, the margin of error is reduced significantly. However, because the incubation period for the AIDS virus can be between two and six months, both tests could fail to indicate that individuals tested had in fact been exposed—the so-called "false negative." False negatives can be as high as 10 percent. Both false positives and false negatives pose major dilemmas.

False negatives can impart to members of high-risk groups, as well as to those with whom they exchange body fluids, a dangerously illusory sense of security. This is one of the drawbacks of the "high-security" singles clubs which are springing up in cities like New York, where membership is contingent on testing negative for the AIDS virus. Who knows whether someone testing negative today and welcomed into the club tomorrow will show up as positive a week hence? How often will tests be required as a condition for membership? False negatives can lull people with multiple sex partners into a perilously false sense of security.

The problem of false positives is just as potentially devastating and damaging. Those who test positive for the AIDS virus are likely to be subject to many forms of discrimination: in employment, in attempting to obtain health insurance, in housing, and, most obviously, in social intercourse. If up to 5 percent of those initially testing positive are, in fact, negative for exposure to the AIDS virus, there is clearly a possibility that many innocent people will be harmed. In light of these facts, ought testing for exposure to the AIDS virus be mandatory or voluntary?

The army has answered this question for the past two years by requiring all recruits to be tested. But the military system is authoritarian, and it is able to insist on uncommonly rigorous standards from its testing laboratories—standards not likely to be upheld by state and local authorities. This will reduce the proportion of false negatives and false positives. Also, those tested by the army are predominantly in low-risk groups.

My own view is that it is both impractical and unethical to require mandatory testing of all citizens. However, mandatory testing of members of certain high-risk groups is worth considering, and voluntary testing of those whose blood is being drawn for other purposes, such as marriage licenses and blood donations, or in the course of receiving ambulatory or hospitalized medical care is to be encouraged.

It seems reasonable, and this is less controversial, that whenever blood is drawn, for whatever purpose, people should routinely be asked for permission to test their blood for exposure to the human immunodeficiency virus. At present, testing is being done extensively without the consent of those from whom blood is being taken. This seems to me to be morally unacceptable. Either the testing for AIDS virus antibodies of blood drawn for other purposes should be mandatory, or else it should be done with the voluntary and informed consent of those concerned. To test surreptitiously is not only deceitful, it also has little value except for either screening out infected donor blood or providing demographic data.

I prefer voluntary to mandatory testing for those whose blood is being drawn for other purposes, but I am willing to concede that a strong case can be made in the interest of protecting the common good by making testing mandatory. If it is mandatory, as is the case now in certain states where those applying for marriage licenses are required to be tested for HIV exposure, then the issues of cost (those being tested are charged up to $300 for the procedure) and waiting time (up to three months to have the test) must be addressed by the state itself.

What is more controversial is to urge the mandatory testing of those in certain high-risk groups. Prostitutes and those convicted of illicit intravenous drug use are obvious targets for mandatory testing. Why, it might be asked, should the members of such groups be singled out? Partly because there is such a high likelihood that many of them will be infected and therefore actively transmitting the disease to others. And partly because those in both groups are engaging in illegal activities. When activities such as prostitution and intravenous drug use threaten the common good, not only because they are inherently destructive but also because they contribute directly to the transmission of a fatal disease, mandatory testing of those engaging in these activities seems a small price to pay in order to reduce this threat.

Reporting Test Results

A related issue is whether or not reporting of those testing positive for exposure to the AIDS virus ought to be mandatory. Here, the key question is, Reporting to whom? It is one thing for the results of a blood test to be made available to public health authorities for the purpose of enabling them to trace and warn those who have had sexual and needle contacts with the individual testing positive; it is another to make these results available to employers, insurance companies, or housing authorities where the possibilities for discrimination are obvious.

To draw this distinction is to reveal my own bias: that reporting to public health authorities in order to protect others is necessary and ought to be obligatory, but that reporting to anyone else might do more harm to the person having tested positive for AIDS antibodies than good to society at large, and ought not to be required. Insurance companies and employers are surely entitled to require tests for exposure to the AIDS virus prior to issuing health insurance or employing personnel. But this does not mean that they are entitled to be informed once an employee or participant in a medical insurance plan has tested positive after the fact.

Adding Insult to Injury

A third question is, Ought the behavior of those testing positive for exposure to the human immunodeficiency virus to be circumscribed—by compulsory tattooing, computerized registration, or quarantining, for example? There are those who argue strenuously that it should. The following is typical of such statements:

> From what we know now the only alternative available until cures or vaccines, or both, are developed, is to prevent the spread of the disease by making it physically impossible. This implies strict quarantine, as has always been used in the past when serious—not necessarily lethal—infections have been spreading. Quarantine in turn implies accurate

testing, which will require the development of an efficient test for viral antigens, not just antibodies. Neither quarantine nor universal testing is palatable to the American public where AIDS is concerned, yet both have been used without hesitation in the past. It is only a matter of time before we, in general, realize that the disease is not peculiar to those with eccentric habits.[14]

That quarantine has been resorted to in the past does not necessarily mean that it is morally appropriate in the present; few would employ this kind of reasoning to support a contemporary slave trade! Further, to quarantine all who test positive for exposure to the AIDS virus would be manifestly unfair to some. There are those—hemophiliacs, for example—who have contracted the disease not as a result of high-risk behaviors but through receiving blood transfusions. Ought they to be quarantined along with prostitutes and intravenous drug users? And, since AIDS is a disease for which there is at present no known cure, to place AIDS victims in quarantine would be tantamount to incarceration for life without any possibility of parole. This seems an outrageously high price to pay, stripping away the civil liberties of some in order to protect the welfare of the many.

Even as I write, there is before me a newspaper headline that reads, "Florida Ponders Locking Up Some AIDS Virus Carriers." A draft policy paper prepared by the Florida Department of Health and Rehabilitative Services proposes that $1.1 million be set aside to commit up to twenty-two adults to a hospital in Lantana and six juveniles to an institution in Orlando formerly used for the mentally retarded. The measure is aimed primarily at prostitutes and others who knowingly expose others to the AIDS virus.[15] Needless to say, the proposal is being widely criticized. The National Gay Rights Advocates condemns it as archaic and as evoking images of the Middle Ages. Nevertheless, it illustrates the as-yet-unresolved tension between individual liberties and the public good.

Another public health proposal is the computerized registration of all who have tested HIV-positive, so that anyone contemplating a sexual encounter can first check out a potential partner. The objections to this should be obvious. A registration system would depend on mandatory universal testing, which must be rejected. Neither registering nor quarantining nor even tattooing—another suggestion seriously propounded by a religious leader of the fundamentalist right—

those who have tested HIV-positive would prevent people who have tested falsely negative from continuing to spread the disease. And computerized registration would make a mockery of any last vestige of confidentiality or privacy the AIDS victim might have. Only in a totalitarian society could such a proposal be taken seriously.

This leads to the conclusion that the best means of ensuring the public good is through tracing those who have had sexual or needle contact with persons with AIDS and urging them to make voluntary behavioral changes so as to reduce the possibility of spreading the disease yet further. Additionally, the general AIDS educational effort must be intensified, beginning at the elementary school level. Prevention remains the best hope for containing the AIDS epidemic. Even if compulsion and coercion were effective means of controlling the spread of AIDS, which, in any case, is dubious, such measures would, in the end, erode values crucial for a democratic society's very survival. This is a price few of us are willing to pay. Voluntary behavioral alteration, based on thorough educational programs, is the only fair and moral way to combat the further spread of this dread disease.

But what about the person who has merely tested positive for the human immunodeficiency virus (HIV), usually but not invariably a precursor to full-blown AIDS? In Chapter 2, we had an example of the cruel choice presented to medical caregivers committed to an ethics in which patient confidentiality is cherished by a young woman who had twice tested HIV-positive and who, nonetheless, continued to have sexual and needle contacts with multiple partners, thereby putting all of them at risk for HIV infection. At present, physicians may not report to the public health authorities cases in which patients have tested positive for HIV, even as they are obliged to report other potentially less lethal venereal diseases or phenomena such as child abuse. This veto on HIV-positive reporting was imposed in California largely because of effective lobbying by the gay community, which justifiably was concerned about possible discriminatory repercussions.

Surely, though, concern for the common good ought to outweigh the patient's right to privacy and confidentiality in a case such as this? Surely, the patient's partners are entitled to be warned against continued contact with the person who has possibly passed on the infection to them and is having sexual or needle contact with others. Surely there is a better way through a dilemma such as this than falsely classifying the woman who tested HIV-positive (not reportable) as having AIDS—so that she could be reported to the health authorities! This was actually done in the case presented in Chapter 2 (see pages 10–11). Under the circumstances, it was perhaps the only responsible course of action open to the medical team. Yet it would have been better for all concerned, the physicians as well as the patient, if HIV had been reclassified as a reportable disease.

Recently, the American Medical Association came out in support of this contention. It recommended that HIV-positive, as well as AIDS, be redefined as a reportable disease, thus representing another warranted exception to the confidentiality standard because of a concern for the general welfare. In states like California, with a highly organized gay rights lobby, translating a recommendation such as this into resolute legislative action will require political integrity and courage of the highest order.

The Socioeconomic Impact of AIDS

Economist Anne A. Scitovsky of the Palo Alto Medical Foundation and her colleague, Dorothy P. Rice of the University of California, San Francisco, have published the most recent analysis of the cost of AIDS, based on 1984 data from the San Francisco General Hospital. The costs incurred by individual patients vary according to their circumstances. Monthly average medical care costs were highest ($3,660) for those patients who died during the year under review, lowest ($586) for previously diagnosed patients who lived all twelve months, and in the intermediate range ($2,617) for those who were diagnosed as having the disease during the year being studied.

Estimates for total national direct personal health care costs of AIDS in 1991 vary from $5.5 billion to $14.5 billion, with a mean of $8.5 billion. This mean figure represents 1.4 percent of all personal health care costs estimated for 1991. By that year, an estimated 5.9 million hospital days will be required to manage AIDS. Furthermore, the advent of new drugs may increase rather than diminish the cost of care: the annual cost per patient of the drug AZT, which can prolong but not spare the life of an AIDS patient, is approximately $12,000.[16]

Who will bear these costs? Jo Ivey Boufford, president of New York's Health and Hospital Corporation, which treats about one-half of all AIDS patients in New York, claims that 70 percent are currently covered by Medicaid, 6 percent by Blue Cross, and less than 1 percent by other commercial insurers. This leaves about 23 percent who are medically indigent.[17] According to another source, the public sector has paid a major portion of the hospital costs for AIDS patients. Approximately 17 percent of the national bill of $380 million for 1985 was paid by private insurance, with public funds paying for most of the remainder.[18] The Medicaid contribution, covering 40 percent of the costs of AIDS treatment in 1985, a sum of $200 million, is expected to increase to $1.8 billion by 1991.

Extrapolating from the present to five years hence, this suggests that by the year 1991, between $1.4 billion and $3.8 billion (a mean of $2.1 billion) of the cost of caring for AIDS patients will not be covered by third-party payers of any kind. Clearly, this represents a societal problem of the utmost magnitude. Only the federal government is in a position to address, let alone resolve, an issue as urgent and as momentous as this. Considering that we already have in the United States approximately 37 million medically indigent persons, and that the present administration has been notoriously tardy in responding to the AIDS crisis, one wonders whether it is not being overly sanguine to expect that the federal government will even begin to mount a response to the economic implications of the AIDS epidemic. Perhaps Peter Carpenter, until recently the Chairman of the Board of the American Foundation for AIDS Research, is right in urging the development of a national AIDS agenda involving the public and private sectors, and the executive and legislative branches.[19] Certainly, this is an issue that ought to be of concern to us all.

So much for the economic projections for the AIDS epidemic, sketchy and tentative as they inevitably are. What about the social impact of this new and fatal disease? Its effect on the single, heterosexual population has been dramatic. Whereas the sixties and seventies inaugurated an era of casual, recreational sexual encounters, the latter half of the eighties has been marked by a return to highly conservative values, characterized by much anxiety and apprehension. Monogamous, stable relationships are being increasingly prized. Marriage, once passé, is again being viewed normatively—even by such mavericks as Hugh Hefner!

Within the male homosexual populations of cities like San Francisco and New York, massive educational campaigns have altered behavior patterns and substantially slowed down the rate at which the disease is spreading. Safer (if not safe) sex is widely advocated and practiced. The gay community itself has played a leading role in this development, assuming much of the responsibility for changing traditional behavior patterns.

Perhaps of gravest concern is the unwillingness, even inability, of intravenous drug users substantially to alter traditional behaviors. Even if free, sterile, disposable hypodermic needles were made available to the members of this community, it is unlikely that this would reduce the spread of the disease. The sharing of needles is not merely a necessity; it has ritualistic connotations as well. The exchanging of blood is a powerful symbol of membership in this in-group. This, coupled with the fact that the will of drug-addicted individuals is inevitably impaired, causes one to be skeptical about the possibility of their being able, even if they were willing, to respond to pleas to change their established behavior patterns.

Of all groups whose members are candidates for having their behavior circumscribed compulsorily in the interests of the common good, intravenous illicit drug users are the most likely. This conclusion does not reflect prejudice against the members of this group; indeed, pity, not prejudice, is my own dominant feeling as I ponder these weighty matters. It does rest on steadily mounting evidence that this is the group most stubbornly impervious to change and most likely to transmit the disease into the wider heterosexual population.

The Risk to Insurers

The American health insurance industry is "a private system with a social purpose."[20] That is to say, it is a private, and primary, means to the end of meeting a major social need: the provision of health care to the people of our country. The industry has always claimed, with some accuracy, that "if it is to be financially viable, creating both relatively broad access to health care and profits for insurance carriers, it must be able to predict with some precision the health care utilization patterns of the insured population."[21] Additionally, it must be able to identify what are called "risk groups": people with similar health service utilization patterns whose average costs can be correlated with insurance premiums.

AIDS presents a direct threat to the principles of sound underwriting upon which the insurance industry is premised. The utilization patterns for people in the general AIDS-related risk group may be disparate to a degree. To test positive for the human immunodeficiency virus does not necessarily mean that a person has AIDS. AIDS and ARC (AIDS-related complex) have different courses. Even among AIDS patients, there are wide differences in the utilization of health services. The case with which this chapter begins is at one extreme; the AIDS patient on a ventilator in an intensive care unit, fighting gamely to the very last, is at the other.

It ought not surprise us, therefore, that health insurance companies, wanting to reduce the risk to their financial viability posed by the phenomenon of AIDS, should come down hard on those likely to be afflicted with the disease—particularly on those newly applying for insurance coverage. Such companies are entirely within their rights to insist on access to medical histories, to examine socio-demographic characteristics, and even to use antibody testing before considering the issuance of a new policy. Unfortunately, this means that "persons who develop AIDS or who consider themselves at high risk for the disease and who do not already have private health insurance are unlikely to find an insurer willing to cover them."[22]

In many ways, the AIDS crisis simply exposes, in a way that is particularly tragic for those already infected or at risk for the disease, the general inadequacies of the American health care system. Throughout this book, frequent allusion has been made to the scandal of our indifference to the principle of distributive justice as exemplified by our enormous medically indigent population. This population will now increasingly include AIDS victims as well as those testing HIV-positive. The blame for this ought not to rest chiefly or solely on the shoulders of insurance carriers. This is a nationwide social problem of the utmost magnitude. Only a resolute response by the federal government will be sufficient to ameliorate it. Thus far, in the Reagan years, the response has been too little and too late. Perhaps the next administration will display more compassion and concern for the powerless and the disadvantaged in our midst. As two commentators conclude,

> perhaps the AIDS crisis, with a predicted cumulative incidence of 270,000 cases by 1991, will rekindle our seventy-five-year-old debate over national health insurance. The expense of this dread disease, if not the ethical considerations of assured access to health care and the broadest distribution of its costs, may drive us as a nation to accept government-sponsored universal coverage. If not, the irony would be that the United States has refused to act upon the one dimension of the AIDS tragedy for which it now has the conceptual solution.[23]

Beneficence Versus Autonomy

We return to the case with which we began this chapter. Gary Davidson had been diagnosed one week earlier as having AIDS. He had been hospitalized eleven days before for a first episode of pneumocystic carinii pneumonia. Now he was refusing the treatment which could probably remedy the pneumonia, but which would not ultimately reverse the underlying disease. He wanted to die now, with dignity, rather than possibly two years later after several bouts of similarly severe illnesses. And he was deemed to be competent to make this decision. Dr. Lois Dorsey and the medical team must decide whether to respect Mr. Davidson's autonomy or, beneficently and paternalistically, to override his wishes and treat him against his will. What ought they to do?

In the previous chapter, in weighing beneficence against autonomy in situations similar to this, I came down on the side of autonomy. However, I added a theological caveat: the prerequisite of attempting to enable a patient to discover or recover a sense of the meaningfulness of life, to be able to look to the future with renewed courage and confidence, and to love and accept love from others.

What was said then bears repeating now. It seems clear that the ultimate obligation of the medical team is to respect Mr. Davidson's autonomous wish to die with dignity. However, their prior duty is to offer help to him in the spiritual domain, facilitating his exploration of faith, hope, and love. More and more, within the network of those volunteers providing support to AIDS patients, their lovers, and their families, there are those whose expertise is in this realm. Often the reason they are experts is that they either have the disease themselves or know intimately people who do. They themselves have had to come to grips with issues of meaning, hope, and love. They are there to help folk like Gary Davidson struggle with these also.

Until this resource has been offered and, if accepted, made available to him, it would be premature simply to accede to his request to die. But neither can he be compelled to accept such an offer. There are limits of decency even to the principle of beneficence. The best solution of this dilemma may lie along the line of striking a bargain with Mr. Davidson: agree for a week to be treated and to have people from the AIDS support network speak with you, and if you still feel after that period of time as you do now, your wishes will be honored.

Patient autonomy is a moral principle most of us have come to cherish. We ought to be able to choose how we shall die, as well as how we shall live. But these choices should be informed. Until Gary Davidson has been informed by those who themselves have had to contend with a diagnosis of AIDS that it is nevertheless possible to live with meaning, with hope, and with love, it would be morally irresponsible to allow him simply to die with dignity in the name of resisting paternalistic beneficence.

A recent study by Bernard Lo and associates at the University of California in San Francisco[24] indicates that an increasing number of AIDS patients are making choices similar to Gary Davidson's. In the early years of the AIDS epidemic, before the ultimate course of the disease was as well understood as it is now, the terminal phase of AIDS was typically managed in intensive care units. AIDS victims would live out their last days and die attached to ventilators, heart monitors, and dialyzers, and with intravenous hydration lines and nasogastric feeding tubes inserted into their bodies. It was not then as clear as it is now that these patients were not salvageable. Now we know that this is the case. According to the principle of salvageability enunciated earlier in this book, intensive care for the end-stage AIDS patient is inappropriate.

What is appropriate is hospice-type care. Lo's study indicates that this palliative approach is more and more being chosen by AIDS patients themselves over the intensive care approach. Even if he was making a premature decision, Mr. Davidson's case is in line with this general trend. It is a trend which I, for one, welcome and applaud as courageous and enlightened to a remarkable degree.

This completes our survey of some of the moral problems being generated by the AIDS epidemic. Of all the issues having to do with the endings of life, this surely is the one presenting twentieth-century medical research and clinical medicine with their most massive challenge. It typically involves young people. Whereas most of us have become reconciled to an acceptance of death at the end of a long and fruitful life, we still feel that the death of young people is an outrage. Something deep within us cries out against it. Yet simply crying out is not enough. Until a cure for this disease is discovered, our responsibility is to prevent its further spread and to enable those who have AIDS to have a compassionate and peaceful death. To these ends, the principle of justice issues an imperious summons to us all.

Retrospect—Why the Issues Proliferate

The field of biomedical ethics is at once fascinating, frustrating, and even somewhat frightening. Fascinating, since it comprehends matters that touch the lives of all of us, one way or the other, sooner or later, for better or for worse. Medicine and the life sciences, and the ethical issues associated with them, exercise an inevitable magnetism over us, whether we are actually engaged in the contest against disease as physicians, allied health professionals, patients, or family members, or as yet are only potentially involved.

For those working professionally in the field, it can be frustrating as well as fascinating. The ethical quandaries generated by medicine and the life sciences multiply at a steadily accelerating rate. Seldom is there a sense of being ahead of the game. Usually one is attempting to catch up with developments that have already taken place, the moral ramifications of which have not yet been fully appreciated. By the time there is a nascent consensus about a morally responsible resolution of one issue, several others have emerged to command attention.

The compelling modern impulse is to put to use new knowledge before it has ripened into wisdom. Our collective capacity to be technologically inventive and innovative threatens to outstrip our moral insight. Not only is it often unclear what ends we are striving to reach, but the means are murky as well. And this gives rise to the nagging fear that we might therefore be led into making some colossal and irreversible mistake, some massive and irretrievable blunder, which would menace the future not only of human life but of all life on this fragile planet.

Of the issues dealt with in this book, only two are still on the horizon—genetic engineering and assisted suicide. They were included because they afford us the rare opportunity to think prospectively about how we might go about handling the developments they portend in ways that will prove to be morally laudable. The other predicaments are already with us. They are presented constantly in the everyday practice of medicine. Nevertheless, a consensus has not yet emerged about morally appropriate responses to them. It is not too late to continue to wrestle with them. If, eventually, thought leads to action, our reflection could contribute to responsible resolutions.

Biomedical ethical issues have proliferated at an astonishingly rapid pace and will continue to do so for at least five reasons.

Technological Innovation

First, there is the phenomenon of constant technological innovation and the tendency to move promptly, if not precipitously, from innovation to application. Bioengineering is an important adjunct to contemporary medicine. In the last fifteen years it has been responsible, for example, for the development of incubators, respirators, and monitoring devices specifically suited to the neonate. Without the advent of these various technologies, neonatology as we know it today would not be feasible. Most recently, the controversial therapy known as extra-corporeal membrane oxygenation (ECMO) has been introduced. In fact, ECMO is really an adaptation of the heart-lung machines which have been used successfully for years in open-heart surgery.

The lively growth of neonatology as a subspeciality of pediatrics led, as we saw in Chapter 8, to a host of ethical dilemmas: When and in what circumstances ought decisions be made to withdraw any technological interventions already instituted or to withhold further interventions? By whom ought such decisions to be made? The parents? The neonatal team? Ethics committees? The courts? Or by those who are footing the bill for this kind of extremely expensive medical care? Ought something like ECMO to be used at all, when it is known that it requires the permanent sacrifice of the artery carrying about a fourth of the blood flowing to the brain? And, with the larger picture in view, ought we to be deploying our relatively limited societal resources on high-cost, high-technology interventions at all, when low-cost, low-technology preventive measures might be more effective in the long run?

Biochemistry is another science fundamental to the modern practice of medicine. Its most profound and important contributions date from as recently as 1962. In that year Francis Crick, a British biophysicist; James Watson, an American biochemist; and Maurice Wilkins, a biophysicist from New Zealand were awarded the Nobel Prize for Physiology or Medicine for helping to determine the molecular structure of deoxyribonucleic acid (DNA), the chemical substance ultimately responsible for the hereditary control of life functions. Since then, several scientists have begun to apply this knowledge to recombine pieces of DNA in order to correct inherent genetic defects—a practice that has come to be known as genetic engineering. Among these are Paul Berg, Stanley Cohen, and Ronald Davis, of Stanford University. Genetic engineering offers the best hope of curing certain inherited diseases, such as diabetes, cystic fibrosis, and many forms of cancer. But it also raises profound ethical questions.

If defective genes can be repaired, either in single cells or in the germ line, then, theoretically, healthy genes can also be enhanced correspondingly, either in single cells or in the germ line. Repairing nonfunctioning or malfunctioning genes may, indeed, be central to the therapeutic enterprise. But, as we have seen, enhancing genes that already function so as to make them perform differently or better raises the specter of eugenics.

If it becomes possible, as one day it might, to enhance the upper body strength of aspiring Olympic gymnasts, the height of basketball players, or the performance of long-distance runners by using the techniques of genetic engineering, then it would also be possible to intervene decisively in the evolutionary process and completely redesign the human species. It is at this point that we move from the realm of technology into areas of philosophy, theology, and ethics. What does it mean to be human? Does our humanity consist merely of the genes we have inherited, or might it also include the genes we can introduce into the pool with our newly discovered techniques? And if we decide to go ahead and reconstitute human nature, who shall draw up the blueprints?

Several additional ethical issues considered in this book have been generated by the phenomenon of technological innovation and application. The new reproductive technologies present dilemmas illustrated by the poignant case of "Baby M" touched on in Chapter 6.

The potential for removing a fetus from the uterus, performing surgery upon it, returning it to the womb, and allowing the pregnancy to proceed to term poses further ethical questions for perinatology. And the technologies commonly applied in the care of adults in intensive care units raise pervasive issues in critical and terminal care which were discussed in Chapter 9. The topics we have thought about in this short volume represent but a small, albeit significant, selection from among the many thrust forward by the development and deployment of biomedical technology.

The Changing Economic Climate

A second factor contributing to the escalation in the number and complexity of biomedical ethical issues is the changing economic climate in which medicine must now be practiced. In 1970 President Richard Nixon warned that the nation was facing a health care crisis because our medical expenditures then amounted to $75 billion (7.5 percent of the GNP). By the end of 1987, health care expenditures in the United States passed the half-trillion-dollar mark: according to the U.S. Department of Commerce and the Congressional Budget Office, our expenditures were $511 billion (11.4 percent of the GNP)[1]. It is clear that something must be done to attempt to curb the inexorable rise in health care expenditures over the past twenty-five years.

Drastic measures were needed if costs were to be held down. These were taken in 1983 by the federal government when it turned away from retrospective reimbursement for actual expenditures in providing hospital care via Medicare to prospective reimbursement on the basis of average costs according to diagnosis-related groups (DRGs). Concomitantly, there has been a dramatic increase in enrollments in HMOs (Health Maintenance Organizations) and PPOs (Preferred Provider Organizations)—all designed to curtail rising medical care expenditures.

Critics of the federal government's expedient point out that the current reductions effect a one-time gain by removing the "fat" from the hospital system, without addressing the persistent underlying factors responsible for the inflation of health care expenditures: costs associated with malpractice insurance, the ordering of unnecessary or repetitive tests; hospitals competing with one another and needlessly replicating services and capital expenditures, and a preoccupation with high technology to the neglect of preventive medicine.

Without entering the debate about the economic merits or demerits of diagnosis-related group systems of reimbursement, it is sufficient for our purpose to point out that they have already created fresh ethical problems for those who practice medicine. Three typical instances are worth mentioning.

One is the conflict set up for physicians by cost-containment systems between their traditional concern to attend primarily to the health of the patient and the emerging necessity to focus also on the financial health of the institutions in which they practice. By way of example, consider the following case from New Jersey, where DRGs were first introduced as a mechanism for reimbursement.

> *An obstetrician-gynecologist at Lakeview Hospital was approached by the hospital's medical director and its director of finance. They pointed out to him that he had admitted seventeen Medicare patients who were later determined to be in DRG 373 (vaginal delivery without complicating diagnosis) but only two in DRG 371 (cesarean section, without complication and/or comorbidity harms inflicted by the treatment). Yet, for the other three obstetricians on staff, fifty-eight of their admissions came under DRG 373 and nineteen under 371. Since DRG 371 afforded the hospital a higher rate of reimbursement than 373, the cost of treating this particular physician's patients exceeded the revenue received from Medicare. Despite his objections that the health of his patients was his primary concern, he was urged to reconsider the way he handled deliveries. The financial health of the hospital, he was told, had to be taken into account as well as the medical health of the patient, since it provided the setting in which individual physicians were able to practice at all.[2]*

Even before incidents like this began to be reported, feminists were becoming alarmed by the fact that delivery by cesarean section was on the increase in this country: one in four babies is now born by cesarean section. Technology was beginning to deprive more and more women of a quintessential feminine experience—natural childbirth. The risk of malpractice liability (extremely high for obstetricians) was one important factor contributing to this trend; now economics further reinforces it.

This introduces a second issue: the growing inability of hospitals working within the constraints imposed by DRGs to provide free care to the medically indigent. Previously, the cost of caring for those who could not pay was spread out among those who could. There were margins within the system for this kind of transference of costs. These margins have disappeared. And the number of medically indigent people multiplies as health insurance companies become increasingly selective about whom they elect to cover.

As has been stated throughout, it is estimated that there are now approximately 37 million Americans who are medically indigent. They are ineligible for federal or state assistance because they are too young or earn too much, yet are unable to afford to purchase private health insurance because they work part-time and do not qualify for company-subsidized benefits, or they work for firms too small to be in a position to offer employees a benefit package. This constitutes a national scandal, surfacing in the medical arena. But ultimately it is a societal rather than a medical concern. Although several economists are working on proposals for the eventual resolution of this problem, no solution is presently in sight. This means that the medically indigent receive short shrift from private and community hospitals. The resources of the county hospitals, their only recourse, are being strained to the breaking point, and the care they are receiving, even in the best of such facilities, is clearly inferior to that afforded those whose costs are covered by health insurance or federal and state reimbursement mechanisms.

A third issue brought to the fore by economic factors is the steady erosion of the commitment by hospitals to care comprehensively for patients, paying attention not only to their physical problems but to their emotional and spiritual needs as well. The ancient Greeks taught us that human beings are an indivisible unity of mind *(nous)*, body *(soma)*, soul *(psyche)*, and spirit *(pneuma)*. Each aspect of our being acts and reacts with and upon the others, which is why one of the more exciting frontiers now receiving medical researchers' attention is that of psychosomatic illness. Many illnesses or maladies are the result of a mysterious conjunction between physical and nonphysical causative factors; migraine headaches and chronic lower back pain are good examples. Precisely what this conjunction is and how it can be reversed is the subject of much contemporary scientific interest.

In the decades following World War II, hospitals had begun to display an increasing commitment not only to meeting the physical needs of those who came to them as patients in terms of procedures performed or medications dispensed, but also to providing emotional and spiritual support and counseling. The importance of enabling people to explore the deep questions of purpose and meaning thrust upon them by their illnesses came to be recognized. Social service and pastoral care departments became institutionalized.

Through these departments, highly trained ancillary health care personnel like chaplains and social workers were accepted onto the health care team and began to work side by side with physicians and nurses in addressing patients' needs in their totality. This vision of comprehensive, or holistic, care and the serious steps being taken to realize it made American medicine exceptional. It represented an enlightened approach to health care of the sort thought possible only within a socialist society such as Sweden, where clergy, social workers, nurses, and physicians alike are employed and deployed by the state.

This vision of comprehensive care, however, is now being threatened by the new systems of cost containment currently instituted and others that might soon be in place. In order to contain costs, hospitals are cutting back on the resources available to social work and pastoral care departments; in some instances, such care is being eliminated altogether. The short-term benefits of this strategy are likely to be more than offset by the long-term costs of the inferior quality of care that will be delivered. In the quest for financial gain, the ideal of humane and holistic medicine could well be lost. If and when this should happen, not only would patients' needs be neglected; those who practice medicine would also be deprived of much that now affords them personal satisfaction and fulfillment, and those who practice allied healing arts would disappear from our institutions.

The Advent of New Diseases

A third factor responsible for the rapid proliferation of biomedical ethical conundrums is the advent of new diseases. In recent memory, several entirely new disease entities have been recognized: legionnaires' disease, toxic shock syndrome, non-A/non-B–type hepatitis, acquired immunodeficiency syndrome (AIDS), and AIDS-related complex (ARC). Of these, AIDS and ARC are the most sinister. In the six years since the human immunodeficiency virus (HIV) was identified, it has generated more ethical quandaries for individuals, health care workers, and society at large than all other diseases combined have done in the previous sixty years. And the end is not yet in sight. Indeed, we have barely seen the beginning. By the year 1992, it is estimated that in the United States alone the cost of caring for people with AIDS will be approximately $16 billion annually, and that AIDS will cost our society approximately $55 billion each year in lost productivity. And this is only one dimension of the problem. Other ethical aspects of the AIDS crisis are steadily emerging, as we saw in Chapter 11.

Changes in the Law

The law itself contributes a fourth factor to the rapid contemporary accretion of biomedical ethical dilemmas. It does so in three ways: in terms of case law; through legislation; and through federal regulations (or attempted regulations).

The cases of Karen Ann Quinlan, Clarence Herbert, Mr. Bartling, Elizabeth Bouvia, Hilda Peter, Nancy Jobes, and Kathleen Farrell (all, with the exception of the well-known Quinlan case, introduced in Chapter 9) had to do with the withholding or withdrawal of life-sustaining intensive care therapies. In three (the Bartling, Bouvia, and Farrell cases) the patients were conscious and competent and were thus able to express their wishes about the discontinuance of aggressive treatment. In the others, the patients were variously described as comatose, in a persistent vegetative state, or irreversibly brain damaged. The decisions to discontinue heroic treatments were made by others—family members, physicians, or the courts themselves. In all of them, the courts either allowed or subsequently upheld decisions to withhold or withdraw mechanical ventilators, and/or intravenous hydration and nasogastric feeding tubes.

These rulings served to settle problems locally. But we see that they created further difficulties if we look at the larger picture. In some cases, the judgments were by county jurisdictions; others were made at the state supreme court level. None is universally binding. In states or counties where no case law precedents exist and where patients' wishes are in conflict with the policies of the medical institutions in which they reside, the traditional state interests—preserving life, preventing suicide, maintaining the integrity of the medical profession, and protecting innocent third parties—will prevail. Inevitably, these will continue to outweigh the right of patients or their surrogates to decide their own fate. Clearly, federal and state legislation is required to establish nationwide, uniform standards of care suited to our present technological capacities.

But legislation itself is not entirely unproblematical. With respect to so-called "right-to-die" legislation, for example, several significant steps have been taken by many of the states in recent years: the Natural Death Act and the Durable Power of Attorney for Health Affairs, both of which have been adopted by a majority of the states, are notable examples. The intention behind each of these pieces of legislation was twofold. On the one hand, they were designed to uphold patient autonomy beyond the point of competence and consciousness. On the other, they were intended to exonerate physicians complying with patients' expressed wishes from all possible deleterious legal repercussions.

But legislative standards in different states remain uneven. We do not yet have in this country a uniform Determination of Death Act consistently defining brain death. In other areas as well, there are not yet in place federally mandated standards applying uniformly across state lines. Besides, each of the pieces of legislation or proposed legislation we have mentioned in the course of this book may be criticized quite specifically. In an area where the precision of the scalpel is often required, legislative measures are frequently blunt instruments. No doubt they will be further sharpened in the course of time.

Federal regulations constitute a third category of legal constraint on the practice of medicine. The purpose of regulations is to protect and benefit patients, especially patients who are particularly vulnerable. Thus, the intent of the so-called Baby Doe regulations was to prevent discriminatory treatment of neonates on the basis of their perceived disabilities, whether actual or probable. And the reason for the Federal Drug Administration (FDA) regulations governing the introduction of new drugs to the market is to safeguard the consumer from undue harm—as happened, for example, when thalidomide was made available before sufficient evidence about its safety had been accumulated through clinical trials.

But good intentions often backfire. The Baby Doe regulations were finally struck down but not before practicing neonatologists had mounted a massive critical assault upon them for being too rigid and not nuanced enough to take account of the complexities of decision making in the perinatal arena. And the FDA regulations prohibiting the premature availability to consumers of potentially dangerous drugs were counterproductive in the case of a drug like AZT, the purpose of which is to arrest the progression of AIDS. The FDA did eventually display unusual flexibility in allowing for its introduction before the standards for controlled clinical trials had been fully met. Other drugs which might be equally useful in the fight against AIDS are still in the course of development. It remains to be seen whether humane considerations will continue to prevail over the inertia of bureaucracy.

Sociological Developments

Finally, a fifth factor contributing to the astonishingly rapid proliferation of current biomedical ethical issues might be termed sociological. What I have in mind as a specific example is the way the nursing profession has now begun to develop and assert its own professional identity, separate from and often putatively in conflict with that of the medical profession. Historically, the nurse was regarded as an extension of the physician. She (even now, 97 percent of all nurses are female) was thought to be there to do the bidding of the physician (until recently, typically male) without qualm or question. Those days are long gone. Nurses now see themselves increasingly as professionals in their own right. They have become conscious of their own unique identity and have declared their own professional standards. These are not always the same as those of physicians. Often, the potential conflict between the two professions becomes actual, as the following case, brought to my attention at a family practice clinic where I conduct a seminar on medical ethics for residents indicates:

One of the patients who appear daily at the clinic is a 23-year-old pregnant woman, the mother of a 15-month-old daughter. The woman's ostensible reason for coming to the clinic each day is that she suffers from migraine headaches, which only injections of Demerol can alleviate. The woman's doctor, partially convinced that she is hypochondriacal but too busy and harried to explore the possible psychosomatic etiology of the headaches, takes the course of least resistance: he writes an order that she should receive injections of Demerol whenever she comes to the clinic. The nurses, who must carry out this order, have a different view of the situation. They are not convinced that the woman's real problem is her headaches; it seems to them that she has become addicted to the Demerol. They have seen her happily playing with her 15-month-old daughter outside the clinic before coming inside, complaining of a migraine headache, for her shot. They suspect that the headaches reflect the state of the woman's marriage rather than her physical condition. And they are concerned about the possible effect on the fetus she is carrying of the powerful drug this woman is receiving each day.

The nurses suggest to the doctor that the woman and her husband be referred to a marriage counselor as a condition for continued medical treatment for her migraine headaches. The physician disagrees. He claims to have explored that possibility before without success. Besides, her insurance will not pay for marriage counseling and the physician himself does not have the time to talk to her about her domestic problems. He argues that the only way to handle this case in a markedly less-than-perfect world is that along which he is currently proceeding. The nurses are outraged. They feel powerless in the face of the doctor's obstinacy. Yet simply to disobey his orders, without being able to prevail upon the woman to explore alternatives, would create more difficulties rather than solve the problem.

This case illustrates the tensions that can and do arise in the practice of medicine between physicians, on the one hand, and nurses as well as other health care professionals such as house officers, social workers, respiratory therapists, and chaplains on the other, as each develops and asserts her or his own professional identity within the health care system. Tensions are being exacerbated by the stresses imposed on all professionals by the economic factors already mentioned. Nationwide, there is a shortage of registered nurses. Hospitals are depending on reduced numbers of nursing and other staff members, even as they attempt to increase both the size and the acuity level of their patient population. Much more is being required of fewer personnel. There is less time for patient care, let alone for the exploration of the subtle ethical issues associated with it. Compliance with physicians' orders on the part of nurses and others saves time; questioning these on ethical grounds and working through the disagreements reasonably and responsibly can be time-consuming. In such a milieu, the ethical quandaries can only become more vexing and intractable.

This completes our review of the various factors—technological, economic, medical, legal, and sociological—contributing to the accelerating number of contemporary biomedical ethical issues. By now, it should be obvious that this is a fertile field for inquiry and debate. But struggling with these issues is more than an academic exercise. It is an urgent necessity for all who practice medicine and for those who work with them side by side, as well as for consumers of medical services. Ultimately, in one way or another, we are all confronted with the responsibility of actually making decisions of momentous import within the biomedical arena, particularly at the beginnings and endings of life. Exercising this responsibility, as was argued in Chapter 1, is not "playing God"; it does not necessarily exhibit grandiosity. It is merely an inevitable concomitant of being human. And humanity, above all else, has to inform and inspire our biomedical endeavors.

13

Prospect—*Quo Vadis*, Medicine?

As we have seen, powerful forces are driving medicine into uncharted moral territory. Precisely where it is going is not yet apparent. Even how many of its present practitioners will continue the journey is uncertain. Older physicians, especially, are retiring from the practice of their art in growing numbers. The life of the physician has become too complicated for them, too fraught with peril, too overburdened with bureaucracy. For the first time in decades, there is a decline in the number of applicants to medical schools. Now that the trapezoid of moral principles has been transformed into a square, juggling the competing claims arising from the four corners—*beneficence, nonmaleficence, autonomy,* and *justice*—has become too daunting and demanding a task. For many, withdrawing to the walnut-growing business or going into financial administration appears to be a more attractive life-style or career choice than playing doctor.

Not only are there likely to be fewer physicians as we look further ahead; in the near term there will be chronic shortages in certain specialties. The number of obstetricians and gynecologists is shrinking, and those continuing in practice are becoming increasingly wary of accepting new patients. Their malpractice insurance premiums are prohibitively high, and the risk of being sued for unfavorable outcomes is pervasive. Similarly, anesthesiology is no longer as desirable a specialty as before, despite its promising financial rewards. Choices about which branch of medicine to practice are being made with a view to minimizing the danger of litigation as much as by wanting to have time for a normal family life.

Hospitals also are in flux. Compelled by the current reimbursement mechanisms to reduce patients' length of stay, hospitals are searching for new programs to increase patient-generated revenue. Some of these succeed, others do not. Same-day surgery centers not only reduce the time patients spend in hospital but are convenient as well. In attracting more patients, these have proved to be a popular and financially rewarding innovation. In contrast, trauma centers, which have also spread prolifically, require elaborate helicopter or fixed-wing aircraft systems to bring patients into the hospital from long distances as well as a wide array of medical specialists, constantly on call, to deal with every conceivable type of emergency. Generally speaking, because they are losing money for hospitals, they contribute to the neglect of the medically indigent.

It used to be the case that questions about how patients intended paying their hospital bills were asked only at the front door upon admission. Those who came in through the back door—the emergency department—were treated first and the question of how the care received was to be paid for was raised only later. Now questions about payment are asked in emergency rooms, often before treatment is provided. If the answers given are not satisfactory, patients may be turned away or sent at some risk and considerable inconvenience to county facilities providing generally inferior care.

At the same time, hospitals more and more are feverishly devising various marketing strategies and emphasizing public relations. Often competitiveness results in superficial rather than substantial improvements—fancy uniforms for those who greet people coming in through the hospital's front door or for those delivering food to patients in their rooms, even as programs essential for the comprehensive approach to patient care, such as social services or pastoral care, are being slashed. Looking good seems to matter more than doing good. What is often forgotten is that public relations efforts are costly and that it is patients or their insurers who end up footing the bill for them. Steadily spiraling *per diem* costs of hospital beds are fueled not only by a falling off in the number of patient days, but also by the sometimes frantic efforts being made to solicit more patients, or "guests," as they are sometimes known—as if hospitals were hotels!

Profound changes on a par with those within the medical profession and the hospital industry are occurring in society as we begin to come to terms with the new economic realities. The latest issue of the *New England Journal of Medicine*, which I have before me as I write, includes an article entitled "The Oregon Decision to Curtail Funding for Organ Transplantation."[1] The opening paragraphs eloquently describe how legislators, as well as physicians, are having to respond to a changing economic climate:

> In the spring of 1987, the Joint Ways and Means Committee of the Oregon legislature faced a painful choice. The Division of Adult and Family Services, charged with administering the state Medicaid program, framed the options for the next two years. During the next biennium—the basic funding period in Oregon—Medicaid could either extend its funding for basic health care to include about 1500 persons not covered previously, or continue to fund a program of organ transplantation (bone marrow, heart, liver, and pancreas) for a projected 34 patients.
>
> In a dramatic example of the type of painful decision necessitated by limited resources, the division advocated the former, and the committee concurred.

The article chronicles the events leading up to this decision, the public reaction to it—the policy "sparked two lawsuits and numerous fundraising initiatives on behalf of those needing transplants"—and the state's response: promising "to reinstate the transplantation program if sufficient private funds could be raised to support it." The authors' conclusion hints at the shape of things to come:

> The message from Oregon is clear: budgetary constraints are real, and they apply to health care. Physicians are welcome to join the debate over choices, but choices must be made. We must look beyond our own vested interest and no longer assume that medicine is any more important than schools, roads, safety, water, or other public programs. Policy makers need our views in order to establish sensible priorities for medical care. If organ transplantation is an important therapy, we ought to help make room for it by suggesting other therapies that are less useful and that can be foregone.

If physicians, hospitals, and legislators are in turmoil, so too is the general public. We spend more on medical care per capita than any other nation on earth, yet our infant mortality rate is as bad as that in some underdeveloped countries! We are the most affluent nation on the planet, yet we have approximately 37 million people in our midst who are medically indigent—to say nothing of our growing homeless population. Our vaunted technological abilities have been called into question as much by our helplessness in the face of AIDS as by the failure of our space program. We want, and in many ways have, the best medical care in the world, made possible by the finest medical researchers and educators, yet growing old in America is terrifying because so few of us can afford the cost of chronic care of the sort provided by skilled nursing facilities and convalescent hospitals, which is likely to consume a lifetime's savings in a matter of months.

Where, then, is medicine heading? Of course, it is impossible to know precisely without benefit of the psychic's prescience. The only certainty is that changes will continue to be demanded and that they will occur, however reluctantly and tardily. It may be possible, nevertheless, to discern some of the areas in which these reassessments and realignments will begin. In concluding, let me suggest five.

The System of Medical Education Will Be Revised

If tomorrow's physicians are to feel at home within the square of moral principles described in Chapter 4, confidently responding to and balancing the competing ethical principles of beneficence, nonmaleficence, autonomy, and justice, then rigorous courses in biomedical ethics will need to be required elements in the medical school curriculum rather than merely electives. In light of the issues we have either mentioned or addressed in this book, that Stanford University Medical School has no full-time faculty member teaching biomedical ethics is unusual. Just 25 percent of my time is funded for this important work, and has been for the past fourteen years.

We should be investing in several full-time faculty members devoted to research and teaching in the field of biomedical ethics. At this particular time, our priorities are to erect concrete structures at a cost of hundreds of millions of dollars. In this respect, our own medical school is not atypical. Although there are some with really fine programs in biomedical ethics, these are exceptional rather than usual. It is clear that this will change in years to come; bioethics research and education will be integrated into the central core curriculum required of every medical student.

Health care economics will be added to the medical school curriculum as well. Already, many of the students who can afford the luxury of a fifth year for medical training rather than the customary four spend much of that year taking courses in the business school. The economic realities affecting medicine are too stark to be ignored. They touch the physician at every turn. There is the cost and the cost-effectiveness of every diagnostic test, from blood tests at a price of hundreds of dollars to magnetic resonance imaging (MRI) scans for a thousand dollars and more.

There are the costs of treatment: procedures ranging from the less invasive to the more invasive, and becoming more expensive accordingly; hospital-based charges; and follow-up and rehabilitative costs incurred after discharge from the hospital. There are convoluted reimbursement mechanisms to be understood and then managed: Medicare, MediCal, Medicaid, DRGs, and other third-party payment systems. There is the cost of malpractice insurance, from tens of thousands to hundreds of thousands of dollars annually, depending on the medical specialty. Like it or not, medicine has become a business. For physicians to succeed, not only as healers but also as managers, the economics of health care will have to become integral to the educational curriculum.

What has been said of the medical student will be true of postgraduate medical education as well, particularly during the years of internship and residency training. Within teaching hospitals, interns and residents, or house staff, as they are commonly known, bear almost all the responsibility for day-to-day patient care while having virtually no authority, as this is vested in the attending physicians. They are the soldiers in the front lines of the war against the ravages of disease and the life-threatening effects of accidents or trauma.

Until recently, they have had little or no help in addressing either the ethical or the economic dimensions of the craft they practice. This too will change. One indication is a recent innovation at Stanford University Hospital: in addition to the 25 percent of my time funded for the teaching of ethics in the medical school, another 25 percent will be devoted to teaching bioethics to house staff in the hospital. This will be done in small seminars with an extensive use of complex case studies elicited from the house officers themselves; actual medical practice will evoke explorations into theory. This development is in step with a nationwide trend in postgraduate medical education.

Hospital Goals: Do Good Rather Than Merely Look Good

During the 1980s, in hospitals throughout the country, there has been a widening of the gap between professed and operative values. Hospitals have professed quality patient care as a dominant value. Several have even had "service excellence" training seminars designed to instill this as a lodestar for all staff attitudes and actions. These programs have been designed to enhance the appeal of hospitals in a competitive market. The goal has been to provide patients and their family members with nurses, physical and respiratory therapists, dieticians, and janitors who are smiling, courteous, obliging, and helpful.

Not just technical expertise is required of hospital workers in the 1980s; just as important is the ability to uphold the values of good public relations. The consumer of medical services is to be regarded and treated as a customer in the same way that the airline and hotel industries view their passengers or guests as customers, to be so coddled and pleased that they will not only make return visits themselves but also spread the word that this particular hospital, rather than that, is the place to come for medical attention.

So far, so good. The catch is that the professed value of service excellence has been subverted at the operative level. Even as programs designed to make the hospital look good have been set in place, behind the scenes the "downsizing" of hospital staff has occurred. Downsizing is a euphemism for either firing employees or reducing them from full-time to part-time status, thus saving the hospital money not only in wages but also in certain benefit payments. The cuts are especially severe in nontechnical areas, in programs that do not directly generate revenue, although they do so indirectly in the goodwill they earn for the institution by affording patients and family members human support, social services, or emotional and spiritual care. Ironically, these are the very departments whose sole raison d'être is doing good—providing disinterested, unconditional counseling and comfort to people undergoing stress.

At the same time, more and more is asked of fewer staff. As hospitals devise new programs to recruit more patients and thus increase patient-generated revenues—for example, trauma centers; bone-marrow, kidney, liver, or heart transplantation units; drug and alcohol rehabilitation centers—so the acuteness level rises concomitantly. Not only are more patients brought in; they are also sicker, more in need of human support, social services, or emotional and spiritual care.

The results are predictable. Staff morale ebbs. "Burnout" becomes more prevalent, particularly, for example, among nurses in intensive care units. Personnel turnover increases. And it becomes evident to everyone except administrators whose gaze is fixed solely on the "bottom line," on profits and losses, that until professed values are reinforced operationally—until hospitals begin again to provide the resources necessary to turn the publicly stated institutional ideal into reality—all public relations endeavors will fail. In the end, superficiality is no substitute for substance.

As we look ahead, this will surely change. The pendulum will swing away from the desire merely to *look* good to the determination to *do* good. Within the next decade, competitiveness will have driven numerous hospitals out of business. Those that remain viable will be compelled to see that many of the cost-saving measures of the 1980s were shortsighted and damaging to staff morale and detrimental to patient care. The vision of caring comprehensively for patients and their relatives will once more come into its own, and there will be the financial commitment to make it possible to attain. Savings in hospital expenditures will be effected. The cuts will come where they have been needed most all along, from reducing the wasteful replication of costly equipment and services, marginally beneficial care, unnecessary tests, and inflated administrative, management, and public relations budgets.

Consumer Expectations Will Be Lowered

This conflict was not perceived during the 1960s and early 1970s or, if it was, it was not thought to be irreconcilable. Americans really did believe then that they could have whatever they wanted, including the moon. The two global oil crises of the mid- and late 1970s, which plunged the world's economy into recession and decline, and the new economic realities affecting medicine in the 1980s have changed this forever. In medical care, particularly, we have been compelled to see that resources are limited and that we cannot have everything we want. Hard, even cruel, choices must be made. As John Kitzhaber, M.D., the Oregon Senate president, expressed it during the debate over discontinuing Oregon's transplantation program:

Is the human tragedy and the personal anguish of death from the lack of an organ transplant any greater than that of an infant dying in an intensive care unit from a preventable problem brought about by a lack of prenatal care?[2]

Whereas understanding the inherent incompatibility between limited resources and unlimited wants is something fairly new for Americans, the citizens of other countries have long been aware of it. In socialist countries like Sweden, allocation decisions are made by the state in light of the resources available and the demographic needs of the population. To a lesser extent this is true in democracies like Britain also. Each of the fourteen regions of Britain's National Health Service allocates the resources with which it has been provided in accordance with the perceived needs of the population within the district. One district will offer open-heart surgery, another will not. In some, neonatal intensive care will be provided, in others not. The difference between Sweden and Britain is that in Britain there is also a thriving and growing private sector. If the wanted surgery is not available in one's district, or the wait for it is too long, one is at liberty to go to Harley Street and have the surgery immediately—at a price.

In the United States, limitations on coverage are already being imposed by federal and state reimbursers and increasingly by private-sector health insurers as well. Underlying these rationing decisions is the tension between the principles of autonomy and justice remarked on repeatedly in this book. Since neither principle is an absolute, autonomy cannot be construed as giving one license to have everything one wants; the common good has to be taken into account as well, in accordance with the principles of distributive justice. Americans will understand this better, even if they like it less, in the decades ahead. Allocation decisions will be made no longer in *ad hoc* fashion, but reasonably, responding to ethical principles, economic realities, and demographic needs. This last will be particularly important. Distinguishing between wants and needs will be the beginning of renewed sanity in the health care system.

Concomitantly, our fascination with high-technology medicine will give way to a belated recognition that it makes better sense to address underlying causes of illnesses than to treat the symptoms after they have arisen. Throughout this book, the point has been reiterated that Americans appear to value high-technology, high-cost interventions over simpler, less expensive preventive measures. Two commentators at the University of Washington offer an explanation of this phenomenon:

> The need for acute care is more visible to the public than the need for preventive care. . . . Acute care commands more media attention than preventive care. Specific people benefit from acute interventions, but it is unclear who will benefit from preventive ones. Also, the benefit of acute care is felt immediately, whereas the benefit of preventive care is realized in the future. A named person who is dying now is more visible than an unnamed person dying in the future. Such unidentified future patients need strong advocates in the medical community.[3]

What the authors left unsaid is that acute interventions cost more than preventive measures. Treating cardiovascular disease by means of coronary artery bypass graft surgery (CABG) is extremely expensive; $10,000 per open-heart operation is commonplace. Educating people to eat less fatty foods, to exercise and lose weight, and to stop smoking is a slower but less expensive expedient. The long-term effects of the surgical and medical approaches cannot be compared. The former saves a relatively few lives and/or ameliorates symptoms, after the fact. The latter prevents cardiovascular disease and enhances the quality of life of far more people at considerably less expense.

Yet the bias in favor of high technology persists and is reflected in the power structure within medical schools across the country. Generally speaking, departments of preventive medicine are "Cinderellas"; their rich stepsisters are the departments of cardiovascular surgery, biochemistry, perinatology, and oncology.

Gradually, the logic of cost-effectiveness will prove irresistible. Probably later rather than sooner, we will come to the realization that it makes better sense, medically and economically, to address the root causes of diseases than it does merely to respond to symptoms.

A Decent Minimum of Medical Care for All

Before the issue of universal health care coverage can be addressed, a prior question has to be raised and dealt with. What does it mean to urge that every American is entitled, as part of the undisputed constitutional right to life, to a decent and necessary minimum of health care? Does it mean *equality of access*—that everyone has the right to be treated in an emergency department without regard for the ability to pay? If this be the case, how far ought treatment to extend? To the high-technology, high-cost interventions we have deplored? Or merely to the point where the patient's condition has been stabilized? Or does it mean *equality of treatment*—that everyone has the right to receive the same treatment as everybody else, no matter how expensive or how little cost-effective? Either way, we come back to the conflict between unlimited wants and limited resources.

Certainly, we mean equality of access. But equally we intend universal health care coverage to denote at least a basic, decent, and necessary minimum; it ought not to reach further than this into the area of unlimited wants, incompatible as they are with shrinking resources. So the question persists: What is this basic, decent, and necessary minimum of medical care to which every American is entitled?

The American Medical Association has begun to take this question seriously. Defining a basic minimum of health care has become one of its urgent priorities. As a consensus builds within the American Medical Association, and as the search for answers is extended to include other bodies representing organized medicine, so concrete proposals will emerge. These proposals will in turn provide legislators with the data they need to subject the ideal of universal health care coverage to the tortuous political process. Eventually, the process will bring forth an ethically acceptable product. Such is the nature—and power—of democracy.

At the same time, proposals for dealing politically with the profound problem of America's 37 million medically indigent people are beginning to emerge. One is that advocated informally[4] by Stanford University's Alain Enthoven. Enthoven's novel solution entails four steps.

First, those presently in receipt of hidden tax breaks on their medical care benefits would accept a ceiling above which they would pay taxes to the federal government. Part of my own salary, for example, presently hidden and tax-exempt, comes to me in the form of the medical care benefits which are provided by my employer, the university, which matches my own monthly medical insurance premiums. All full-time employees of companies and corporations throughout the country with medical insurance benefits are similar beneficiaries of hidden, tax-exempt salary increments.

Second, a payroll tax of a few percent would be levied by the federal government on small businesses which, because of their size, are currently unable to offer their employees medical care or other benefits. The revenues generated by this small-business payroll tax would augment those accruing from the tax on above-the-ceiling employee benefits.

Third, each state would provide basic medical care to all its residents, to be subsidized in part by the federal government from the tax revenues in the two categories mentioned above. Above-the-ceiling medical care benefit tax revenue, augmented by the payroll tax on employers not now furnishing their employees medical care benefits, would be returned by the federal government on a pro rata basis to the states, so that they, in turn, could partially subsidize their own decent and necessary minimum medical care entitlements.

Fourth, the recipients of medical benefits within each state would be expected to contribute a small proportion of the cost of the medical care they receive. The states' programs would be subsidized by the federal government and paid for in part by individual recipients of medical care benefits. There would be no free lunch. For most of the medically indigent, this would be entirely acceptable. Remember that the medically indigent population is not comprised of those who are unemployed. The unemployed or the unemployable would continue to be taken care of as they are now, by federally mandated programs.

As was explained earlier, the majority of the medically indigent are part-time employees, eligible neither for benefits from their employers, who provide benefits only to their full-time employees, nor for federally funded programs like Medicaid, which provide for the unemployed. Others work for companies too small to be able to offer their few employees medical and other benefit packages. Most of the medically indigent are women in their late twenties or early thirties, single heads of households, with small children. The fact that they are responsible parents wanting to work part-time rather than full-time in order to be with their children causes them to be discriminated against when it comes to benefits provided by employers.

This, in broad outline, is Enthoven's approach to the pervasive problem of medical indigence in the United States. The details must be filled in and further refined. Even then, whether or not the proposal is accepted in Washington in January of 1989 will depend largely on the then presidential incumbent and the political party in power. This means that it cannot now be predicted when the time for this idea will be seen to have arrived. The idea itself, however, has its own intrinsic merit and appeal. Sooner or later, probably later, it will be translated into a program of universal health care coverage.

The Malpractice Phenomenon

I n her book, *Defective Medicine: Risk, Anger, and the Malpractice Crisis*, Louise Lander has a chapter headed "From Unhappy Patient to Angry Litigant."[5] It begins with the following story:

> The medical press was triumphant; on June 1, 1976, after over a year of nothing but disaster to report on the malpractice front, a victory had finally been scored on the side of the medical profession. A doctor sued for malpractice had the guts to sue his patient back, and a jury in Chicago had found the patient, her husband, and her lawyers liable for "wilful and wanton involvement in litigation without reasonable cause" and the lawyers also liable for legal malpractice.

Such satisfying moments for physicians are few and far between. They are also more than outweighed by the costs to consumers of malpractice litigation. However exorbitant physicians' malpractice insurance premiums may be, it is not they, but we, who in the end foot the bill. We do this both directly and indirectly. Directly, the consumer pays because whatever it costs physicians to insure themselves against malpractice litigation is simply passed on to patients in the form of inflated charges or to patients' insurers who, in turn, raise their premiums. Indirectly, consumers, or their insurers, pay because physicians practice medicine defensively, with an eye to possible later legal repercussions. This means that they order unnecessary and often extremely costly diagnostic tests and embark on elaborate and sometimes inappropriate therapeutic regimens ineffective relative to costs in order to protect themselves should their patients later prove unsatisfied and sue.

There is not the slightest doubt that this peculiarly American phenomenon (other developed societies are notably less litigious) contributes significantly to the constant escalation of the cost of medical care. If costs are to be contained in the interests of our being able to provide a basic and necessary minimum of health care services to all our citizens, the malpractice system of redressing consumer grievances will simply have to change.

Changes will occur on two fronts. One is that the medical profession will begin to monitor the performance of its members more closely, and those physicians discovered to be practicing incompetently or inappropriately will be swiftly and rigorously disciplined. In the past, peer review mechanisms have been too lax. Impaired or incompetent physicians have not been adequately reviewed and dealt with by their colleagues. The fairly recent case of the anesthesiologist at a well-known medical center in the University of California system comes to mind.

This individual practiced oral sex with his anesthetized female patients over a period of several years without his colleagues observing, let alone protesting, his behavior. When his case was finally brought to light, it was due to the action of a laboratory technician who noticed high concentrations of sperm in the fluids suctioned from the mouths of the anesthesiologist's female patients! One would have thought that in their own—to say nothing of their patients'—best interests, the surgeons would have been concerned to observe an anesthesiologist's operating room exploits and have taken the steps necessary to put an immediate stop to such flagrant patient abuse. But no. Somehow this doctor's nearest colleagues were oblivious to his totally unprofessional conduct.

There are such things as patient neglect and patient abuse. Impaired and incompetent physicians do practice medicine. They bring no credit either to themselves or to their profession, and they constitute a real and present danger to the public. This in large part accounts for the malpractice phenomenon in the United States. Unhappy patients do become angry litigants. Inevitably, this will change. To the extent that the medical profession is itself uneasy with the current malpractice climate, it becomes more willing to practice constant, disinterested peer review, followed, where necessary, by immediate disciplinary action. The economic realities circumscribing medical care can only serve to reinforce this trend.

On a second front, there will be a move away from malpractice litigation as a means of redressing consumer grievances to some system of arbitration. Consumers are surely entitled to compensation for physical and emotional pain and suffering resulting from medical mismanagement or mistakes. This no one would wish to deny. But that these compensatory damages should be inflated because contingency-fee malpractice lawyers stand to gain as much as 33 percent of awards in successful suits borders on the obscene. The voracious appetite of contingency-fee lawyers, as much as the impaired or incompetent physician, is to blame for the current malpractice crisis surrounding medical care. This will have to change, giving way to a system of arbitration between aggrieved consumers and the providers who inadvertently caused them damage.

This completes our attempt to predict the shape of things to come. One response to the question *Quo vadis*, medicine? has been ventured. It expresses the need for change in at least five important areas:

- The whole system of medical education will be revised;

- Hospitals will come back to a concern to do good, rather than wanting merely to look good;

- Consumers of medical services will lower their expectations and come to terms with the fact that there is an irreconcilable conflict between limited resources and unlimited wants;

- Leaders of the medical profession and the legislative branch will agree on what it might mean to provide all Americans with a decent and necessary minimum of medical care;

- Malpractice litigation as a means of affording recompense to consumers for legitimate grievances will eventually be supplanted by a better system, perhaps that of more rigorous peer review coupled with arbitration.

This sounds like a wish list. Perhaps it is. But it also represents my own deepest convictions about the necessity for changes in the practice of medicine, the areas where these are needed most, and our ability to rise to the challenge. Only the medical profession, the hospital industry, legislators, and the general public *together* can make a difference. In years to come, whether or not medicine evolves into a more or less humane enterprise for patients and providers alike will depend on how well we all manage to collaborate in responding to the problems that have been identified.

Even though several shortcomings in the present system have been identified and needed changes suggested, there are times when an imperfect system works almost perfectly. This is certainly to be seen in our final case. In spite of inadequacies in medical education, the financial constraints experienced by hospitals, the unrealistic expectations of many consumers, the ongoing problem of medical indigence, and the risks of malpractice litigation, an ethically courageous and compassionate decision was made in this case.

Chen-Yu, a 19-year-old student at Berkeley, was found by one of his four brothers lying in a pool of blood on the bathroom floor. It appeared that he had shot himself in the head, but was not quite dead. His brother called the paramedics, who arrived promptly and transported Chen-Yu to the nearest hospital. In the emergency room of Washington Hospital, the patient received six units of blood, was placed on a breathing machine, and was then transferred immediately to Stanford University Hospital because of his extensive self-inflicted injuries.

On admission to our intensive care unit, the patient's status was found to be as follows. Chen-Yu, intending to kill himself, must have flinched as he pulled the trigger of his handgun; instead of blowing his brains out, he had completely severed his spinal cord, leaving himself utterly paralyzed from the neck down. He had also almost entirely removed his palate, esophagus, and tongue; if he survived, years of reconstructive surgery would be required for him ever to speak or swallow. The massive blood loss he had sustained before being found by his brother had caused apparently major brain damage. He was also medically indigent: no longer covered by his parents' health insurance policy; covered by his student health policy for only minor illnesses; and ineligible for MediCal or Medicare coverage because he was a student working part time.

Communicating with Chen-Yu's family, who spoke only Chinese, proved challenging. Fortunately, one of the doctors in the intensive care unit was married to a Chinese woman and had considerable knowledge of the family's culture—a necessity in situations of this nature for which his medical education had not prepared him. And a volunteer in the hospital's chaplaincy department spoke the family's dialect fluently (volunteers and private donations have helped keep the chaplaincy department strong despite financial cutbacks). Through the volunteer, the family—Chen-Yu's mother and father, his four brothers, his uncle, and his grandmother—unanimously communicated to the care team their wish that Chen-Yu's life not be sustained heroically by artificial means and that he be allowed to die quietly.

Since it was too early to know the extent of Chen-Yu's brain injury, the team deferred any final decision until the neurologists were able to assess his mental status over a period of at least three days. The family agreed to wait for a series of neurological tests to be performed. If the patient proved to be brain damaged, but not brain dead, allowing him to die could be legally hazardous: it was both illegal and risky from the perspective of possible malpractice litigation later.

Although Chen-Yu was medically indigent, the hospital was willing to absorb the considerable cost of caring for him. The hospital's administration felt that no other facility in the area could provide Chen-Yu with the specialized care he needed, and that having agreed to admit him for medical reasons, it would be unethical to discharge him because of financial considerations.

Throughout the next three days, Chen-Yu was maintained in a stable but critical condition and the family remained unanimous in their wish that his existence not be prolonged artificially. At the end of three days, the neurological team confirmed everyone's worst fears: Chen-Yu was not brain dead; he was extensively brain-damaged and would never again be capable of independent living. If he survived, he would need to be placed permanently in an institution. Had his injuries been sustained before he turned 18, the lifetime cost of Chen-Yu's institutional care would have been borne by the state. Since he was 19 years old, this cost would have to be borne by his family; it was a potentially catastrophic situation for them financially. With these facts, the intensive care team and the family together made the decision not to increase the medications necessary to maintain Chen-Yu's blood pressure; this meant that his blood pressure steadily dropped until he quietly died, while still connected to his breathing machine.

Since Chen-Yu's death was a result of an apparent suicide attempt, the county coroner had to be summoned. It was entirely possible that when the medical records revealed that the immediate cause of death was the decision not to increase the medication necessary to maintain Chen-Yu's blood pressure, all those who had been party to that decision, myself included, would be subpoenaed. It was also remotely possible that some other member of Chen-Yu's family who had not been involved in the decision-making process could later file a malpractice suit against the hospital. We assumed these risks because, under the circumstances, we felt that the decision made was entirely appropriate. Chen-Yu had been suicidal for about eighteen months. He had bought his handgun a year previously. He had seriously intended to kill himself. We felt that if he had not wanted to live with a whole mind and body, he would certainly not have wanted to live completely paralyzed, profoundly mentally impaired, unable to breathe without a machine, and incapable of speaking or swallowing. The decision made honored both his wishes and those of his family. It also demonstrated the moral integrity of the hospital and the intensive care team.

Notes

Chapter 1

1. Paul Ramsey, in *Ethics at the Edges of Life* (New Haven: Yale University Press, 1978), frequently refers to physicians playing God. See, for example, pp. 203ff.
2. This point is discussed throughout a scholarly yet readable book by Victor R. Fuchs, *How We Live: An Economic Perspective on Americans from Birth to Death* (Cambridge: Harvard University Press, 1983).
3. Genesis 2: 16b–17.
4. Genesis 3:12.
5. Genesis 3:14.

Chapter 3

1. The Tarasoff case (*Tarasoff vs. Regents of the University of California*) established a legal precedent which now provides one notable exception to the standard of confidentiality. The court held that it is the physician's duty to breach confidentiality in order to warn someone whose life is being threatened by a potentially dangerous psychiatric patient.
2. The writings ascribed to Hippocrates (circa 420 B.C.) are all deontological in nature.
3. *Dictionary of Medical Ethics* (New York: Crossroad, 1981), p. 263.
4. As examples of the duty of nonmaleficence, consider *Romans*, 12:17, 21, and *Matthew*, 5:44–46, 47b–48.
5. Two recent books illustrate the difficulty of defining what is meant by justice as a guiding principle. These are: Karen Lebacqz, *Six Theories of Justice* (Minneapolis: Augsburg Publishing House, 1986), and Robert M. Veatch, *The Foundations of Justice* (New York: Oxford University Press, 1986).
6. The parable of the prodigal son (Luke 15:11–32) is a paradigm of the principle of autonomy. Although the father in the story does not particularly like the behavior of either of his sons, he respects their need to act out their Oedipal conflicts in order to arrive eventually at maturity.

Chapter 4

1. *Salgo* (1957), followed by *Gray* (1966), *Berkey* (1969), and *Cooper* (1971), all reinforced the view that not to obtain from a patient or subject an informed and voluntary consent constitutes a battery.

2. *Natanson v. Kline* (1960) is the landmark case in which not to inform is equated with negligence.
3. *Canterbury v. Spence* (1972), *Cobbs v. Grant* (1972), and *Wilkinson v. Vesey* (1972) all serve to unite battery doctrine with a negligence theory of liability.

Chapter 5

1. This matrix is presented by W. French Anderson in "Human Gene Therapy: Scientific and Ethical Considerations," *The Journal of Medicine and Philosophy*, vol. 10, no. 3, August 1985, pp. 275–291. I am indebted to Mr. Anderson for many of the ideas developed in this chapter.
2. W. French Anderson and John C. Fletcher, "Ethical Issues in and Beyond Prospective Clinical Trials of Human Gene Therapy," *The Journal of Medicine and Philosophy*, vol. 10, no. 3, pp. 293–309.
3. W. F. Anderson and J.C. Fletcher, "Gene Therapy: When Is it Ethical to Begin?" *New England Journal of Medicine,* 303, 1980. pp. 1293–96.
4. W. F. Anderson, "Human Gene Therapy: Scientific and Ethical Considerations," ibid., p.281.
5. Ibid., pp. 282f.
6. Ibid., p. 283.
7. Ibid., p. 285; Anderson raises this question forcefully here.
8. Ibid., p. 288.
9. Philip H. Rhinelander, *Is Man Incomprehensible to Man?* (Portable Stanford, Stanford Alumni Assn., 1973).
10. Cf. Leslie Stevenson, *Seven Theories of Human Nature* (New York: Oxford University Press, 1973).
11. Marc Lappe, "Eugenics: Ethical Issues," *Encyclopedia of Bioethics*, vol. 1, ed. by Warren T. Reich (New York: The Free Press, 1978), pp. 466f.

Chapter 6

1. *Report of the Committee of Inquiry into Human Fertilization and Embryology,* chaired by Dame Edith Warnock, Department of Health and Social Security (London: Her Majesty's Stationery Office, July 1984), p. 4.
2. Cf., for example, Mark S. Frankel, "Reproductive Technologies: Artificial Insemination," *Encyclopedia of Bioethics*, vol. 4 (New York: The Free Press, 1978), pp. 1444–45.
3. This figure is based on current costs and success rates at clinics such as that in New Norfolk, Virginia.
4. Even if the legalities of this case were undisputed, I would want to continue to draw a clear distinction between morality and the law. What is legal may not necessarily be moral; what is moral may not inevitably be legal.
5. *Instruction on Respect for Human Life in its Origin and on the Dignity of Procreation: Replies to Certain Question of the Day,* submitted by Congregation for the Doctrine of the Faith (St. Paul Edition, February 1987), II, B: 4, p. 289.
6. Ibid., p. 46.
7. Ibid., p. 47.
8. *Report on the Disposition of Embryos Produced by In Vitro Fertilization,* presented by Committee to Consider the Social, Ethical and Legal Issues Arising from In Vitro Fertilization (Melbourne, State of Victoria, Australia, August 1984).

9. *The Ethics Committee of the American Fertility Society, Ethical Considerations of the New Reproductive Technologies*, Sept., 1986, vol. 46, no. 3, *Fertility and Sterility*, Supplement 1.

10. Ibid., p. 63S.

11. Ibid., p. 67S. The committee does nothing to enlighten us as to how it expects this interesting clinical social experiment to be conducted.

12. Ibid., p. 46, italics added.

13. Ibid., p. 46.

Chapter 7

1. The pro-life group includes the hierarchy of the Roman Catholic church and many of the church's members, the so-called moral majority (right-wing fundamentalist Protestants), and atheists like Bernard Nathanson, whose views are eloquently propounded in *Aborting America* (New York: Doubleday, 1979). It is worth nothing that "in the Jewish community today, with a conscious or unconscious drive to replenish ranks decimated by the Holocaust, contemporary rabbis invoke not the more lenient but the more stringent Responsa of the earlier authorities. The more permissive decisions, they point out, were in any case rendered against the background of far greater instinctive hesitation to resort to abortion. Against today's background of more casual abortion, rabbis are moving closer to the position associated with Maimonides and Unterman, allowing abortion only for the gravest of reasons," David M. Feldman, "Abortion: Jewish Perspectives," *Encyclopedia of Bioethics* (New York: The Free Press, 1978), p. 8.

2. The pro-choice group includes liberal Protestants and lay or religious Roman Catholics, feminists, secular humanists, and philosophers such as Michael Tooley. Tooley's landmark article, "Abortion and Infanticide," *Philosophy and Public Affairs*, vol. 2, no. 1, Fall 1972, in which he adopts a developmental view of human nature, shows him to be favorably disposed to both abortion and infanticide on the grounds that neither the abortus nor the neonate have yet developed to the point where they possess a serious right to life—something Tooley reserves for self-conscious persons only.

3. Distinguished representatives of the mediating positions are Sissela Bok, "Ethical Problems of Abortion," *Hastings Center Studies*, Jan. 1974, vol. 2, no. 1, and Jane English, "Abortion and the Concept of a Person," *Canadian Journal of Philosophy*, Oct. 1975, vol. 5, no. 2. Preeminent in this group is Daniel Callahan, *Abortion: Law, Choice, and Morality* (New York: Macmillan, 1970).

4. These data are presented and then interpreted in one-sided fashion by Bernard Nathanson in a purportedly documentary film entitled *The Silent Scream*.

5. Cf. John T. Noonan, Jr., "An Almost Absolute Value in History" in *The Morality of Abortion: Legal and Historical Perspectives*, ed. John T. Noonan (Cambridge: Harvard University Press, 1970), pp. 51–59.

6. Cf. Beverly Wildung Harrison, *Our Right to Choose: Toward a New Ethic of Abortion* (Boston: Beacon Press, 1983).

7. James M. Gustafson fairly characterizes the syllogistic form of the argument in his essay, "A Protestant Ethical Approach," in Noonan, *Morality of Abortion*, op. cit., pp. 102ff. As Gustafson points out, this argument is typically made from an external viewpoint by persons who claim the right to judge the actions of others. They confine their arguments to physical factors, excluding moral and spiritual concerns. They tend to deal almost entirely with the patient and physician at the time of the particular pregnancy, omitting other relationships and a larger time frame. They assume that

the natural law position from which they reason is universally compelling and binding—even on persons who do not share their religious stance.

8. "Whereas the God-given inviolability of the conceptus at every stage is the central affirmation of abortion opponents, several related arguments usually are put forward. One is the contention that a principal mark of a just and compassionate society is its defense of the defenseless, its special concern for the weak and the powerless—in this case surely the fetus. Of all living beings involved in a contemplated abortion, it is only the fetus that cannot speak for itself and thus needs to be surrounded by special legal and moral protection," James B. Nelson and Jo Anne Smith Rohricht, *Human Medicine* (Minneapolis: Augsburg Publishing House, 1984), p. 52.

9. The argument is that permissive legal attitudes to abortion have the consequence of protecting the life and health of women (physically, mentally, and emotionally) and that restrictive abortion laws have the opposite result.

10. Cf. Ernlé W. D. Young, "An Approach to the Teaching of Biomedical Ethics," *The Monist*, vol. 60, no. 1, January 1977, pp. 121–135.

11. In the second trimester, "medical evacuation of the uterus seeks to emulate the natural mechanisms of labor and delivery at term by initiating uterine contractions, thereby dilating the uterine cervix and expelling the uterine contents. The initiation of contractions is induced by injecting into the amniotic fluid a concentrated solution of salt or twenty-five to forty mg. of a hormone called prostaglandin. . . . The former tends to kill the fetus, while the latter does not." André E. Hellegers, "Abortion: Medical Aspects," *Encyclopedia of Bioethics*, vol. 1, p. 4. To avoid difficulties for the woman aborting, as well as for those performing the abortion, urea is commonly injected into the amniotic sac when prostaglandin is the preferred means of initiating contractions, to ensure that the abortus is delivered dead.

12. Cf. Ernlé W. D. Young, "Improved Imaging Techniques May Nudge Abortion Debate to the Right," *Diagnostic Imaging*, Sept. 1984, pp. 44–45.

13. Frank A. Chervenack, M.D. et al. "When is Termination of Pregnancy during the Third Trimester Morally Justifiable?" *New England Journal of Medicine*, vol. 310, Feb. 23, 1984, pp. 501–504.

14. "Improved Imaging Techniques," p. 45.

15. Cf. Ruth R. Faden and Tom L. Beauchamp, *A History and Theory of Informed Consent* (New York: Oxford University Press, 1986).

Chapter 8

1. *Deciding to Forego Life-Sustaining Treatment: Ethical, Medical, and Legal Issues in Treatment Decisions*, report of President's Commission for the Study of Ethical Problems in Medicine and Biomedical and Behavioral Research, March, 1983. (Reprinted by Concern for Dying—An Educational Council, 250 W. 57th St., NYC 10107).

2. Nancy K. Rhoden, "Treating Baby Doe: The Ethics of Uncertainty," *Hastings Center Report*, vol. 16, no. 4, August 1986, pp. 34–42.

3. Cf. Ann Burns Gerraughty and Linda J. Younie, "ECMO: The Artificial Lung for Gravely Ill Newborns," *American Journal of Nursing*, May 1987, pp. 655A–658F.

4. Op. cit., p. 663.

5. Cf. Jeff Lyon, *Playing God in the Nursery* (New York: W.W. Norton, 1985) and Rasa Gustaitis and Ernlé W. D. Young, *A Time to Be Born, A Time to Die* (Menlo Park, CA: Addison-Wesley, 1986).

Chapter 9

1. Substantial parts of this chapter were published in "Life and Death in the ICU: Ethical Considerations," by Ernlé W. D. Young, Ph.D., Chapter 6 of a textbook edited by Joseph M. Civetta, M.D., Robert R. Kirby, and Robert W. Taylor, M.D., entitled *Critical Care* (Philadelphia: J.B. Lippincott, 1988). I express my gratitude to Joseph M. Civetta, M.D. for his permission to use material from this chapter in the present volume.
2. Cynthia B. Cohen, "Ethical Problems of Intensive Care," *Anesthesiology*, 17.2, August 1977, pp. 217–227.
3. *Critical Care Medicine, National Institutes of Health Consensus Development Conference Summary*, vol. 4, no. 6, 1983.
4. Two recent books illustrate the complexity of arriving at any consensus about the meaning of the term. They are Karen Lebacqz, *Six Theories of Justice* (Minneapolis: Augsburg Publishing House, 1986) and Robert M. Veatch, *The Foundations of Justice* (New York: Oxford University Press, 1986).
5. 163 Cal. App. 3d 190, 209 Cal. Rptr. 220.
6. The President's Commission for the Study of Ethical Problems in Medicine and Biomedical and Behavioral Research, *Deciding to Forego Life-Sustaining Treatment: Ethical, Medical, and Legal Issues in Treatment Decisions*, March, 1983.
7. William Winkenwerder, Jr., M.D., "Ethical Dilemmas for House Staff Physicians," *Journal of the American Medical Association*, Dec. 27, 1985, vol. 254, no. 24, pp. 3454–57. Cf. the editorials in the same issue of JAMA, "Moral Disagreements During Residency Training," and "Doctor's Orders," pp. 3467–68.
8. 147 Cal. App. 3d 1006, 195 Cal. Reptr. 484.
9. Barber and Nejdl v. Superior Court, 147 Cal. App. 3d 1006, p. 1011.

Chapter 10

1. Substantial parts of this chapter were originally presented by the author at a national conference entitled "Assisting Suicide: The Legal, Medical, and Ethical Issues," at Stanford University, April 2–4, 1987. Entitled "Assisted Suicide: An Ethical Perspective," it was subsequently published in *Issues in Law & Medicine*, vol. 3, no. 3, Winter 1987, pp. 281–293. I am indebted to the editor, James Bopp, Jr., J.D., for his permission to include it in this volume.
2. From the introduction by Derek Humphry, Executive Director of the National Hemlock Society, to *A Humane and Dignified Death: A New Law Permitting Physician Aid-in-Dying*, by Robert L. Risley (Glendale, CA: Americans Against Human Suffering, 1987). Americans Against Human Suffering sponsored an initiative to legalize physician-aid-in-dying in California.
3. Immanuel Kant argued in his *Groundwork of the Metaphysics of Morals* that human beings ought always to be treated as autonomous ends and never as means. John Stuart Mill speaks of the individuality of action and of thought in his celebrated treatise, *On Liberty*. What Mill means by liberty is similar to what Kant denotes by autonomy.
4. Tom L. Beauchamp, "Paternalism," *Encyclopedia of Bioethics*, ed. Warren T. Reich (New York: The Free Press, 1978), pp. 1194–1201.
5. The 1980 edition of the *Statistical Abstract of the United States* reveals that suicide ranks among the top five causes of death for white males aged 10–55, and is the second-ranked cause of death for all males aged 15–24. Nearly 30,000 Americans choose to

end their own lives annually; many experts believe that the official statistics grossly understate the actual number of suicides, perhaps by half.

6. Figures are for 1984.

7. "Generally, perons who use the most lethal methods in their suicide attempts and are unsuccessful have a lower risk of future suicide attempts than do those who use the less lethal methods. In other words, the person who survives a self-inflicted gunshot wound is less likely to try suicide again than someone who unsuccessfully used a plastic bag," Lynne Ann deSpelder and Albert Lee Strickland, *The Last Dance: Encountering Death and Dying* (Palo Alto: Mayfield Publishing, 1983), p. 364.

8. The negative psychological, emotional, spiritual, physical, and sociological effects of suicide on survivors are steadily being substantiated.

9. The point that suicide often follows in the wake of a profound loss of meaning is made by Robert Kastenbaum and Ruth Aisenberg in *The Psychology of Death* (New York: Springer Publishing, 1972), p. 251.

10. H. Tristram Englehardt, Jr., *The Foundations of Bioethics* (New York: Oxford University Press, 1986), p. 306.

11. The Hemlock Society was founded in 1980. It supports the options of active voluntary euthanasia for the terminally ill and assisted suicide. Hemlock's "Guide to the Self-Deliverance of the Dying" is entitled, *Let Me Die Before I Wake*, published by the Hemlock Society, P. O. Box 66218, Los Angeles, CA 90066. "Exit" is the British equivalent of the Hemlock Society.

12. Donald M. Wright, "Criminal Aspects of Suicide in the United States," *North Carolina Central Law Journal*, vol. 7, no. 1, Fall 1975, pp. 156–163, carefully describes three aspects of the criminality of suicide: the act itself, attempted suicide, and the act of a second person aiding or encouraging the suicide. For general background, as well as a specific state-by-state analysis of laws regarding suicide, attempted suicide, and assisting suicide, see Marzen et al., "Suicide: A Constitutional Right?" *Duq. Law Review*, 1, 17–100, (1985) pp. 148–242.

Chapter 11

1. *The Hastings Center Report*, vol. 4, no. 1, February 1984, "If I Have AIDS, Then Let Me Die Now!" a case study by Sophia Vinogradov et al., pp. 24–26.

2. *The Hastings Center Report*, vol. 17, no. 3, June 1987, Abigail Zuger and Rose Weitz, "Professional Responsibilities in the AIDS Generation," pp. 16–23. See also Abigail Zuger and Steven H. Miles, "Physicians, AIDS, and Occupational Risk," *Journal of the American Medical Association*, vol. 258, no. 14, Oct. 9, 1987, pp. 1924–28. See also James R. Allen et al., "A Special Supplement—AIDS: The Responsibilities of Health Professionals," *Hastings Center Report*, vol. 18, no. 2, April/May, 1988.

3. *The Hastings Center Report*, vol. 16, no. 6, December 1986, "AIDS: Public Health and Civil Liberties," a special supplement by Deborah Jones Merritt et al.

4. *Health Affairs*, vol. 6, no. 3, fall 1987, "Update: Socioeconomic Impact of AIDS," by John K. Iglehart, J. Leighton Read, and James A. Wells, pp. 137–47.

5. *The Hastings Center Report*, vol. 16, no. 5, October 1986, Gerald M. Oppenheimer and Robert A. Padgug, "AIDS: The Risk to Insurers, The Threat to Equity," pp. 18–22.

6. Anne A. Scitovsky, "The Economic Impact of the AIDS Epidemic on U.S. Health Resources," unpublished paper presented at a Health Services research seminar at Stanford in Dec. 1987.

7. *The New York Times*, Nov. 13, 1987, p. 10.

8. *Report on the Council on Ethical and Judicial Affairs: Statement on AIDS*, Dec. 1, 1986, Office of the General Counsel of the American Medical Association.

9. *Current Opinions of the Judicial Council of the American Medical Association* (Chicago: The American Medical Assn., 1984), p. xi.

10. Robert Wachter, "Sounding Board: The Impact of the Acquired Immunodeficiency Syndrome on Medical Residency Training," *The New England Journal of Medicine* 314 (1986), pp. 177–180.

11. Abigail Zuger, *The Hastings Center Report*, op. cit., p. 19.

12. Alasdair MacIntyre, *After Virtue* (Notre Dame, Indiana: University of Notre Dame Press, 1981).

13. Abigail Zuger and Steven H. Miles, *Journal of the American Medical Association*, op. cit., p. 1927.

14. James F. Grutch, Jr. and A.D.J. Robertson, "The Coming of AIDS," *The American Spectator*, vol. 19, March 1986, p. 15.

15. *The New York Times*, Jan. 27, 1988, p. 10.

16. John K. Iglehart, J. Leighton Read, and James A. Wells, "The Socioeconomic Impact of AIDS on Health Care Systems," *Health Affairs*, vol. 6, no. 3, Fall 1987, pp. 142–43.

17. Ibid., p. 143.

18. Dennis Andrulis et al., "The Provision and Financing of Medical Care for AIDS Patients in U. S. Public and Private Teaching Hospitals," *Journal of the American Medical Association*, 11, Sept. 1987.

19. John K. Iglehart et al., ibid., p. 147.

20. Gerald M. Oppenheimer and Robert A. Padgug, "AIDS: The Risks to Insurers, the Threat to Equity," p. 19.

21. Ibid., p. 19.

22. Ibid, p. 20.

23. Ibid, p. 22.

24. Robert Steinbrook et al., "Preferences of Homosexual Men with AIDS for Life-Sustaining Treatment," *New England Journal of Medicine*, vol. 10, no. 7, Feb. 1986, pp. 457–60.

Chapter 12

1. Eli Ginzberg, "A Hard Look at Cost Containment," *New England Journal of Medicine*, vol. 3l6, no. 18, April 1987, pp. 1151–54.

2. Jeffrey Wasserman, "The Doctor, the Patient, and the DRG," *Hastings Center Report*, vol. 13, no. 5, Oct. 1983, pp. 23–25.

Chapter 13

1. H. Gilbert Welch and Eric B. Larson, "The Oregon Decision to Curtail Funding for Organ Transplantation," *New England Journal of Medicine*, vol. 319, no. 3, July 1988, pp. 169–171.

2. John Kitzhaber, "Who'll live? Who'll die? Who'll pay?" *Oregonian*, Nov. 29, 1987, B1, B6.

3. Welch and Larson, op. cit., p. 173.

4. Prof. Alain Enthoven's proposals for dealing with our national problem of providing medical care to the indigent were outlined in one of my medical ethics classes at which he spoke in the spring of 1988.

5. Louise Lander, *Defective Medicine: Risk, Anger, and the Malpractice Crisis* (New York: Farrar, Straus, & Giroux, 1978).

About the Author

Ernlé Young was born in Johannesburg, South Africa. He received his B.A. in Systematic Theology and Biblical Studies and his Master of Divinity in Systematic Theology from Rhodes University in South Africa. An ordained minister of the United Methodist Church, he and his family first came to the United States in 1967. In 1971 he received his Ph.D. in Theological Ethics and Systematic Theology from Southern Methodist University in Dallas.

In order to work for social change, in 1971 he returned to Bloemfontein, South Africa, the most conservative part of the country, as Superintendent Minister responsible for 42,000 Methodists—most of whom were black, others of mixed race, and yet others white—and as pastor of the 1,500-member Trinity Methodist Church.

He became extensively involved in attempting to reform the apartheid system, within the church as well as in the political arena. In pursuit of this goal, he founded in Bloemfontein a branch of the Progressive Party, the only political party in South Africa committed to an integrated society.

In 1973 he learned that he was to be banned by the government for these activities and left South Africa while there was yet time. He came to Stanford at the beginning of 1974, to develop a Chaplaincy Department in the hospital and to initiate the teaching of medical ethics in the Medical School. He is presently Chaplain to the Medical Center and an Associate Dean of Memorial Church.

Author of many articles, Ernlé Young is also co-author of a book entitled *A Time to Be Born, A Time to Die: Conflicts and Ethics in an Intensive Care Nursery,* published by Addison-Wesley in 1986. He and his wife Margaret have four children. His hobbies include furniture making, long-distance running, backpacking, tennis, jazz, and photography.

Index